375

A REPLY TO IVAN ILLICH

**This book is to be returned on or before
the last date stamped below.**

HOLIDAY LOAN

-5 FEB 1986

819104.

HORROBIN

MEDICAL HUBRIS

A REPLY TO IVAN ILLICH

DAVID F. HORROBIN

CHURCHILL LIVINGSTONE
EDINBURGH, LONDON AND NEW YORK 1978

F EME

CHURCHILL LIVINGSTONE
Medical Division of Longman Group Limited

© David F. Horrobin 1977

This edition © David F. Horrobin 1978

First published by Eden Press, Montreal,
Canada 1977
Published by Churchill Livingstone 1978
    Reprinted 1979

ISBN 0 443 01814 6

British Library Cataloguing in Publication Data
Horrobin, David Frederick
  Medical hubris.
  1. Social medicine
  2. Illich, Ivan
  I. Title
  301.5   RA418   78-40394

Printed in Hong Kong by
Wah Cheong Printing Press Ltd.

Preface

Ivan Illich's books on medicine have made a considerable impact. They have not yet been subjected to sustained and detailed criticism from within the medical profession. *Medical Hubris* is an attempt at such a critique.

Illich has written two books on the same theme. The first, *Medical Nemesis — The Expropriation of Health*, was a paperback which achieved a wide circulation in many countries. The second, somewhat expanded version was called *Limits to Medicine*. The chapter headings and sub-headings and most of the references in the two versions are identical.

On the whole I do not dispute the facts which Illich has culled from the literature. I have therefore quite deliberately not engaged in a reference slogging match by quoting large numbers of my own. I am happy to accept most of his sources. What I do dispute is Illich's interpretation of these facts and it is the argument about interpretation which is the main theme of *Medical Hubris*.

Those readers who have already read *Medical Nemesis* or *Limits to Medicine* will undoubtedly get most out of *Medical Hubris*. My chapter titles, headings and sub-headings are the same as his with the exception of the last chapter in *Medical Hubris* which has no parallel in the Illich books. Each section of my book refers to the section with the same title in the Illich books. The reader who has one or both of the Illich books can therefore readily identify the passage to which I am referring. All the Illich quotations in *Medical Hubris* are taken from *Medical Nemesis* although most of them also appear in *Limits to Medicine*.

However I also wanted to make *Medical Hubris* a book which could be read straight through in a profitable manner even in the absence of the prior reading or ready availability of one of the Illich books. At the beginning of each chapter or section I have therefore tried to summarise as fairly as possible what I think Illich is saying. I have tried to make his views and mine clearly separate.

Practising doctors and busy medical scientists are often impatient with those who are interested in the underlying philosophy of medicine. They accept the Conventional Wisdom of the Dominant Group (contracted to the acronym COWDUNG by the late C.H. Waddington in his outstanding book, *Tools for Thought*) that we do not have to fuss about philosophy.

They are wrong. Philosophy may take a long time to work through the system but what we are doing today frequently reflects the philosophy of the leading thinkers thirty, forty or fifty years ago. Illich's philosophy is currently influencing many people. If doctors do not analyse that philosophy, accepting it where it is right and opposing it where it is wrong, in thirty years' time they may find themselves the unwilling practitioners of a system which reflects the working through of Illich's ideas.

I think Illich is important. I think he is influential. I think he is sometimes right. But more often he is tragically wrong. It would be a disaster if his views became widely accepted by medical planners simply because they have not been adequately analysed. *Medical Hubris* is an attempt at such analysis.

Montreal, December 1977   D.F.H.

Statement by Marion Boyars Publishers Ltd.

The material quoted from Ivan Illich's MEDICAL NEMESIS — THE EXPROPRIATION OF HEALTH is taken from the original publication which appeared as a draft or working paper in the *Ideas in Progress* Series in 1975. The *Ideas in Progress* Series draft, which is now out of print, was subsequently revised and re-written and published under the new title LIMITS TO MEDICINE: MEDICAL NEMESIS — THE EXPROPRIATION OF HEALTH by Marion Boyars Publishers Ltd., London 1976. Readers are advised that the definitive version was restructured and re-written by the author in response to a world-wide reaction to the original draft which was published in many languages including French, German, Dutch, Swedish, Norwegian, Spanish, Serbo-Croatian, etc and the definitive version is available in these and many other languages besides.

Marion Boyars
May 9th 1978

Contents

A*

1 Introduction

'The medical establishment has become a major threat to health.' So opens Ivan Illich's brilliant polemic *Medical Nemesis*. I agree. I agree with many of the other things Illich says in his profoundly disturbing and stimulating book. But, I sharply disagree with many others. Illich hankers vaguely after some ill-defined past Utopia when things were different and better. He combines this rueful backward look with a determinist approach to the future in which only two scenarios are possible, one bright, the other disastrous.

In a few places Illich demonstrates considerable ignorance of medicine and the medical world. But examples of this ignorance are few and I was surprised not by the occasional error but by the amount of knowledge. The emphasis is overwhelmingly on the situations in Mexico and the United States and some of the extrapolations to other parts of the world are certainly unjustified. Illich's possible answers to the problems he describes are over-dramatic and highly unlikely to be realised. They go so much against what most people seem to want that they could never be achieved in democratic countries. On the other hand, they so strongly emphasise individual freedom that it is hard to imagine them being permitted under any totalitarian regime. A country ruled by that mythical figure the benevolent dictator would seem to be the only place where Illich's ideas could be put into practice. And as I shall try to demonstrate that seems to me to be Illich's failure. He is one of Plato's Guardians, a clever, good man who knows what the people need but is unwilling to take undue notice of what they might want.

I read *Medical Nemesis* with much enjoyment, occasional irritation and a growing sense that this could prove one of the key medical documents of the second half of the twentieth century. It seemed to me that a substantial and detailed reply from the medical profession was required, a reply which frankly acknowledged where he was right and was constructively critical where he was wrong. I felt that if the medical profession took up the challenge to serious debate then great good might be done. I have been disappointed by the response. The weekly medical journals did their best and some devoted a good deal of space to synopses of the book and to reviews. Most reviewers were relatively impressed with Illich although a few were petulantly superficial. A few writers irrelevantly concentrated their attacks not on the arguments but on the man and supposed discrepancies between his life style and his philosophy.

Since then the silence in the medical world has been deafening. As far as I am aware there has been no detailed reply to Illich from within the profession. Almost incredibly most doctors I talk to seem still to be ignorant of his existence. Most of those who have heard of him are unremittingly hostile — often without having read *Medical Nemesis*. Many of those who do know what Illich is saying seem to be hoping that if the profession keeps quiet the man will be discouraged and go away, and not need to be taken seriously. Such doctors forget that medicine is now nowhere very securely in the hands of the profession (Illich would naturally rejoice at this). Laymen now make many of the decisions which shape the medical future and may be very receptive to at least some of Illich's concepts. 'There is nothing so practical as a good idea' as Mr. Brezhnev recently stated at the 25th Congress of the Communist Party of the Soviet Union. Some of Illich's ideas are very good, some are very bad, but almost all are brilliantly expressed and to the uninformed layman they may all sound equally convincing. Illich's ideas are going to penetrate medical politics whether the profession likes it or not. It would be unfortunate if even the good ones were not put into practice without full and rigorous debate.

Despairing of replies from other doctors, I have decided to write this book as a contribution to what I hope will be a critical, constructive and long-continued debate about our current medical problems and their future answers. It would be a tragedy if Illich's ideas were put into practice unchanged. It might be an even greater tragedy if they were ignored by the profession and allowed to die.

Since the opinions expressed in books like these are inevitably shaped by personal histories, I think an author should be obliged to provide at least a brief autobiography. Readers may then be able to provide explanations for particular views and blind spots. Some of Illich's difficulties seem to me to be related to his personal experiences of particular members of the medical profession in particular parts of the world. I think it is important that readers should be able to identify the origins of my own idiosyncrasies.

I was brought up in two industrial towns in Northern England, Bolton and Blackburn. My first experiences of the medical profession were entirely favourable. I was exposed to two 'old-style' family doctors who were supreme examples of the type. The first was an elderly Scot. My father had been his first baby delivered in general practice. I was the first baby of that first baby and the object of particular attention and gruff kindness. The second, a Lancastrian, was of my father's generation and a close family friend. He played in the cricket team for which I kept score. Between the ages of 10 and 13 I frequently went with him on his rounds and learned what a doctor's devotion to the interests of his patients could be. Later, as a medical student, I returned to him for my time in general practice and he has remained a close personal friend. It was he who stimulated my desire to go into medicine.

I went to Balliol College, Oxford to read medicine and entered a quite different sort of medical world where research was the dominant influence. All medical students then had to do an honours degree in physiology. The purpose of this was to teach the basic science of medicine and to provide the opportunity for one to learn to think. At Balliol I came under the influence of Sandy Ogston, one of the most remarkable of Oxford tutors. He understood very clearly the difference between teaching and learning so brilliantly described by Illich in *Deschooling Society*. At my first tutorial he stressed that I was the only meaningful judge of what lectures and practical classes were of value to me. He said that I must make up my own mind as to what I found valuable and that on no account should I waste my time by going to formal courses which to me seemed to have little merit. I regret to say that I found very few of value and Sandy expended much effort in successfully defending my viewpoint against a number of irate teachers. I spent four idyllic years during which weeks often went by without my attending a single lecture or laboratory class. But I did read and I did have to discuss every week with Sandy or some other tutor what I had read. The comments were often scathing and gradually I learned to be critical and to think for myself.

While at Oxford I also learned to travel. During my second year at Balliol I was awarded a remarkable travel scholarship provided by W.A. Coolidge of Boston, an ex-Balliol man. Each summer he took eight Balliol undergraduates across the Atlantic and provided each with transport and ample funds to enable him to travel anywhere in the United States and Canada. For four months of a memorable summer, I roamed the North American Continent from Boston to Vancouver, from San Francisco to Key West. I learned how limited my geographical horizons had been. I also learned how surprisingly different from what I had known in Britain medical practice was in the U.S.A. In innumerable discussions I clarified my concepts of the relative merits of the two traditions.

My desire for travel, stimulated that summer, has since proved near insatiable. The following year I spent four months in Africa. Most of this time I spent working for an embryo flying doctor and mobile medicine service based in Nairobi in Kenya. I criss-crossed the country seeing the surprising sophistication of the capital, the possibilities for African development revealed by the rich farmlands and the problems and the delights of almost untouched tribal communities. Two years later I again left Europe to lead an expedition to the Himalayas whose aim was to plot blood group patterns among the peoples of Nepal.

In 1969, after completing my medical studies at St. Mary's Hospital in London and doing my internship at a small market town general hospital in Northern England, I returned to East Africa to become Head of the Medical Physiology Department in the new Nairobi Medical School. In my spare time I wrote *A Guide to Kenya and Northern Tanzania* and in order to do this dragged my long-suffering family to remote corners of both countries. I observed at first hand the contrasts between the Kenyan and Tanzanian approaches to development, with Kenya determined to pull at least Nairobi into the 20th century high technology medical system at almost any cost and Tanzania taking a much more critical view of the value of modern hospital medicine. In 1972 I returned to England to teach for three years in the Newcastle University Medical School. In 1975 I moved to Canada, to the Clinical Research Institute of Montreal where I am almost exclusively concerned with laboratory research on medical problems.

My attitudes to medicine and medical education have without doubt been heavily influenced by my years at Oxford. In spite – or because – of my somewhat cavalier attitudes to formal tuition, I did relatively well and soon after receiving my honours degree in physiology was awarded a Fellowship at Magdalen College. Magdalen is perhaps the most medically distinguished of all Oxford colleges. Five Nobel prize winners (Sherrington, Robinson, Florey, Medawar and Eccles) had taught or studied there and I was fortunate enough to meet the last three. There was a constant stream of distinguished medical visitors who over dinner appeared to treat me as an equal and expected me to talk with them on their own terms. I inevitably became fascinated by medical research. This has been my dominant concern over the years. However, this concern with research has constantly been tempered by my early experience with outstanding family doctors, by my exposure to the medical problems of the developing world and by the intense satisfaction I obtained from doing my internship in a small general hospital with no research programme. I am interested in opening up the medical profession to people with a wider range of social and intellectual backgrounds than at present enter it and I have played an active role in trying to get medicine established as an appropriate subject for the Open University in Britain. I am concerned with the reactions of patients and relatives to the medical enterprise and I have been involved with the British Schizophrenia Association. This organization, primarily consisting of relatives of patients, has been trying to obtain more sympathetic understanding both among health professionals and among the lay public for people with this disease. I have little doubt that many of the arguments I present will be seen as idiosyncratic. I hope that this brief autobiography will enable readers to identify at least some of the origins of my personal views.

Since the specific purpose of this book is to reply to Illich's *Medical Nemesis*, I have imposed upon myself the structure of his work. I have attempted to answer him chapter by chapter, to acknowledge freely where I think he is right, to criticize uncompromisingly where I think he is wrong and to make constructive alternative suggestions of my own.

There is no doubt that the state of medicine is unhealthy. Illich has brilliantly.and on the whole accurately described the syndrome. But his understanding of the causes of the sickness seems to me to be largely defective. Because of this his prescription for treatment, if followed, will lead to disaster.

2 The Epidemic of Modern Medicine

Illich starts with the fact that in Western society the pattern of disease and death has changed dramatically over the last 100 years. Infections have largely been eliminated as killers except in the elderly, the newly born and the debilitated. This change is commonly attributed to the impact of modern medicine. Illich claims that medicine has contributed almost nothing to the changed pattern, that modern medical care has insignificant effects in the treatment of disease and that modern medicine actually damages health in major ways. Illich believes that to tackle the problem by reforming medical care systems is futile: only a revolution offers any hope. For Illich these points are 'obvious, well-documented — and well-repressed'.

It is foolish to deny that there is substance to each of these charges. Some doctors who are rabidly anti-Illich have unfortunately displayed their foolishness. But in almost every situation Illich overstates his case and in some he presents a view which to the uninformed must be frankly misleading. Each of the points made is considered carefully in the following sections of the chapter. In this introduction I shall draw attention to two crucial general matters.

In forty-five footnotes to the chapter Illich draws attention to about 60 books or articles containing the information which provides the basis for his work. The great majority of these books and articles was written by serious members of the medical profession and published by mainstream medical publishers or major medical and scientific journals (for example, the *British Medical Journal, Science, Journal of the American Medical Association, Canadian Medical Association Journal, American Heart Journal, American Journal of Medicine, New England Journal of Medicine* and *Pediatrics*). In no sense can these be considered radical or fringe publications. They are the major 'establishment' journals of the profession. Most of the evidence on which Illich's polemic is based has therefore been gathered by doctors concerned about the problems of their own profession and anxious to improve the situation by bringing them into the open. This evidence has then been freely published in the important journals respected by most doctors. It is exceedingly unlikely that any other profession (certainly not the law) would be as openly self-critical and as careless in the publication of damning evidence. In this area at least medicine may perhaps be the most forward looking of all the professions.

Having said that, it must also be said that while the evidence has not been repressed, it has most certainly been ignored by most doctors. The impact on medicine of many of the studies quoted by Illich has been negligible. Articles have been published but not read. Cogent criticism has not been taken to heart and has led to reform neither of attitudes nor of practice. Illich has performed a major service by demonstrating just how strong is the case for the prosecution.

The other general point I wish to make concerns Illich's use of the terms *significant* and *insignificant*. These are key words of his, repeated many times in the argument. Yet at no point is it clear to the reader without specialist knowledge what Illich means by them. The word significant can be used in a statistical sense where it has a precise and specialised meaning which I shall enlarge upon later. It also has its common non-technical meaning of *important* (the Shorter Oxford Dictionary says of significant 'full of meaning or import, important'). Throughout the chapter Illich uses the word in its technical, statistical sense. Throughout he gives the impression that he is hoping that lay readers will take it as having its ordinary meaning. This leads to gross misrepresentation.

One of the functions of statistics is to give some indication as to whether a particular event may have occurred by change or whether it may be attributed to some direct cause. By employing a variety of techniques which need not be considered here, statistics can be used to assess the impact of a particular course of action. Suppose there is a disease which long experience has shown to kill about half the people who suffer from it. In a particular outbreak, twenty people with the disease are given the old ineffective treatment and twenty are given a new treatment of unknown efficacy. In the former group, the expected ten individuals die whereas in the latter, only eight die. In this case a statistical analysis of the situation shows that such a result in the group given the new treatment could occur in a group given the old treatment more than once in twenty such trials. The result is therefore said to be 'not significant' in a statistical sense. Conventionally the cut-off point for statistical significance is the 1 in 20 level. If an event could occur by chance more than once in twenty trials, the outcome is usually said to be statistically not significant. If it could occur by chance less than one in a hundred times, it is 'statistically highly significant'.

Significant in the technical sense is merely an expression of probability. It gives no measure whatsoever of the *importance* of a particular event. Importance is a relative concept which has little meaning unless it is made clear to or for whom or what a particular event is important. If my child dies within a week of being born, it is an event of supreme importance for myself and my wife. It is of major but rather less importance for my parents and brothers and sisters. It is of moderate importance to my friends, of slight importance to my acquaintances and of no importance at all to those who know nothing of me. In another sense the death of that child may be important to a wider circle if its illness gives clues as to the reasons for death in a much larger group of infants. In Donne's sense it is of importance to all humanity, 'Ask not for whom the bell tolls ...'. But few of us are capable of carrying consciously the immense burden which that attitude implies.

In no sense is the death of that child alone statistically significant. One extra infant death will normally make no difference to the analyses of infant deaths in the hospital, in the city or in the country. In a statistical sense the death is non-significant (the statistical expression) or to use the incorrect expression employed by Illich it is insignificant. In a human sense the death of that child is of supreme significance, certainly to myself and to my immediate family and depending on attitudes, perhaps to a much larger circle as well.

It is essential not to mix the statistical and ordinary uses of the word significant. When used in its ordinary sense of important, it is necessary to define or to imply for whom the event is or is not important. When used in its statistical sense in a publication for laymen it is only honesty to make clear that it is not being used to mean important. It is also essential not to employ statistical methods which are frankly misleading and to clarify the nature of the question being asked using the statistical technique.

Consider a rare disease like muscular dystrophy which affects perhaps one in every three thousand individuals born. Few individuals with the disease live a normal span and many die young. Suppose that these premature deaths were eliminated. Suppose one were then to ask whether this dramatic change had a statistically significant effect in extending the average life span of human beings. The disease is so rare that of course the answer would be that the treatment had a statistically non-significant — or to use Illich's term — insignificant effect. The question is of course silly. The question which should be asked is whether the treatment extends the life span to those to whom it is administered, namely those with muscular dystrophy. In this case the effect of the treatment would be statistically highly significant.

If one were to ask whether such a treatment of muscular dystrophy were important, there could only be one answer. By all the things which make us human such an event *must* be important. It would be important primarily to the victims and their families but also in a real sense to anyone capable of understanding what the disease means.

Illich consistently uses the words significant and insignificant in the irrelevant statistical sense of whether treatment of a particular disease has an impact on the health of a whole population. Equally consistently he uses the words in contexts which to the uninitiated suggest that they have their common meaning. It is difficult to know whether or not the confusion is conscious or not. Either way it is a major source of the power of Illich's writing in this chapter. If the confusion is removed many of the arguments lose much of their force.

Doctor's effectiveness – an illusion

Illich claims that 'the specifically medical treatment of people is nowhere and never significantly related to a decline in the compound disease burden or to a rise in the life expectancy'. Provided that the word significantly is used in a strictly statistical sense, provided that the statistics are used to answer the rather silly sort of question illustrated by asking whether a complete cure of muscular dystrophy would extend the average life span of the whole population and provided that the expression 'specifically medical treatment' is very narrowly defined, Illich is right. The great changes in the patterns of disease are primarily related to changes in the environment, in the nutritional status of a population, in the supply of clean water and in the effective disposal of excreta. The major killing infectious diseases in most cases declined in importance long before they were completely understood or specific medical treatment became available.

But Illich misrepresents the story. Many of the important environmental changes, particularly in the supply of clean water, the safe disposal of excreta and the provision of specific items of diet such as iron and vitamins, were initiated and put into effective use by doctors. In many cases it was doctors who were stimulated and provoked by their contact with disease, who saw the relationships between nutrition, water supply, sanitation and illness, and who forced authorities to take action. If one follows the history of any of the great killers one finds a story of intense argument and bitter confusion among the medical profession, with a myriad of causative factors being proposed. Out of that confusion came slow improvements, a decline in the effectiveness of the disease and greater understanding. Sometimes greater understanding led the way, sometimes a purely empirical event produced a decline before understanding came. Either way the understanding was important in ensuring the permanence of the decline. A lively interest on the part of the medical profession was almost always important in creating an appropriate atmosphere for advance, even when the eventual causes of the improvement proved not to be specifically medical. Similarly most thinking doctors feel that the modern epidemics of heart disease, of cancer, of ulcers will decline as a result of measures which are not specifically medical. But these measures will emerge out of and be understood because of the intense intellectual interest in these matters on the part of the medical profession.

The work which led to the control of the infectious diseases has become so incorporated into our Western way of life that its origins have been largely forgotten. But because of this failure of memory it is inexcusable to deny that the medical profession played a key role in controlling many though obviously not all of the killers. Similarly, there can be little doubt that heart disease, cancer, arthritis, diabetes and mental disturbances are largely environmental in origin. But the precise environmental problems which are the roots will not be discovered without the probing of doctors using modern research techniques. And when that happens, the diseases will decline in importance and their medical treatment will be a problem confined to small numbers of people. But to say that the medical profession plays no part in changing disease patterns just because the method finally effective in controlling the disease is non-medical is nonsense.

Illich makes much of the truism that most of modern medicine consists of a struggle to handle disease which cannot yet effectively be prevented or treated. It is only from this struggle that the new insights will emerge which will enable the disease to be largely taken from the medical realm.

The expression 'specific medical treatment' is used by Illich in a rather peculiar sense. When using it, he means only those measures which can be employed exclusively by those with a full medical training. Other measures which can be used by those without a full medical training are excluded. In this way Illich eliminates from the medical realm vaccination and immunisation, the use of hygienic techniques by midwives and the widespread use of certain antimicrobial drugs such as the anti-malarials. This seems to me to be the most special sort of special pleading. All these measures and others like them were developed as the result of research by doctors and without the medical profession would almost certainly not exist.

It is when he discusses the infectious diseases that Illich's confusion of the statistical with the common meaning of the word significant is particularly likely to lead to gross misunderstanding. Illich may be right when he claims that in Western countries the medical prevention of the deaths of children and young people from such diseases as pneumonia, appendicitis, malaria and typhoid fails to have a statistically significant impact on the life expectancy of the population as a whole. This is hardly surprising because partly as a result of past medical research most people in Western societies do not experience these illnesses and most people live until old age. But the appropriate question to ask is not 'Does medical intervention in childhood pneumonia significantly increase average life expectancy of the total population?' but 'Does medical intervention increase the average life expectancy of that small part of the population which develops pneumonia in childhood?' The answer to the first somewhat trivial question is no whereas that to the second much more important one is yes, even in a statistical sense. And only someone with a lack of true understanding or with a debased concept of humanity would deny that the lives saved are important. They are important first to those immediately concerned and second to the community as a whole in giving confidence that these former killers of children can now be effectively controlled. One does not need to read many nineteenth century novels before one begins to appreciate just what that confidence means.

Illich says that new treatments of pernicious anaemia, hypertension, haemophilia and congenital heart disease redefine but do not reduce morbidity. Again in one sense he is right. This was not understood by the pioneer architects of the British National Health Service who believed that once medical care was available to everyone, illness would go away and the need for such care would be substantially reduced. It is still not understood by many intelligent people both inside and outside the medical profession. If the total amount of morbidity experienced during the lifetime of an individual is considered, then unless one is made both immortal and immune to all disease, the longer one lives the more disease one will experience. There are two reasons for this. First since certain common events such as colds and minor injuries occur with relatively constant frequency throughout life, the longer one lives, the more of them one will experience. Second, the killing diseases of the young tend to do their work rapidly while those of the old are frequently long and drawn out. The longer one lives, the more pain and illness one experiences. In this sense if modern medicine saves individuals from an early death, it is not only redefining morbidity but actually increasing it.

In another and to me much more important sense Illich is simply being silly. He seems to be implying that it is better to die early as the result of a stroke than to live a much longer if mildly uncomfortable life as a result of treatment for hypertension: it is better to die young because of pernicious anaemia than to live a long and in this case virtually normal life as the result of modern treatment with injectable vitamin B_{12}: it is better to suffer crippling illness for a few years as a child with congenital heart disease than it is to be cured as a result of open heart surgery.

Illich's view is in a long and academically respectable tradition. The idea that it is better for the young to be killed quickly in their prime is a favourite one among poets and churchmen comforting their relatives. 'Whom the gods love die young', 'Not lost but gone before', 'They shall not grow old as they that are left grow old', are sentiments which have been repeated again and again and again. They rarely sound convincing to the close relatives of the dead. One suspects that to most of the dead themselves they would sound very hollow indeed. G.A. Studdert Kennedy, affectionately known as Woodbine Willie, perhaps the greatest of all war chaplains, adored by the soldiers in the trenches of the Somme because he always had a friendly but realistic word for everyone, expressed my view precisely:

> *For comfort and for love of God*
> *Deliver us from cant.*

Illich may genuinely believe that the only thing we are doing when we cure pernicious anaemic or congenital heart disease is to redefine mortality without reducing it. He may even find a few doctors and laymen to agree with him. But I suspect that most ordinary people with a grain of common sense would dismiss him with little more than a rude gesture.

Useless medical treatment

Illich claims that in the past medical treatment saved few lives and that today the situation is no better. He concedes that in a few infections such as gonorrhoea, syphilis, malaria, yaws and pneumonia, modern chemotherapy can be effective. But because in these situations chemotherapy is relatively inexpensive and easy to apply, he implies that it does not come into the realm of 'specific medical treatment' and therefore cannot be put down to the credit of the medical profession.

Illich claims that drug treatment of tuberculosis, tetanus, diphtheria and scarlet fever has played a 'minor, possibly insignificant role' in the total decline in morbidity and mortality from these diseases. Once again he is largely correct but is so at the expense of being seriously misleading. To say that lives saved by therapy of malaria or tuberculosis are not significant is again to confuse a technical statistical term with its common use. To deny that immunisation against tetanus and diphtheria are medical measures because they are frequently administered by those who are not doctors is once more misleading.

Illich is right when he says that medical successes against non-infectious diseases have been less convincing than those against the infections, but he is blind to the few real successes. He writes that 'replacement therapy lessens the direct impact of diabetes, but only in the short run'. Thus to dismiss one of the most dramatic of medical advances, the discovery of insulin, and its use to save lives which were literally flowing away, displays a less than generous attitude and a failure to give credit where credit is due. The truth is that there are undoubted problems about the long-term control of diabetes. The truth is also that many young people who would otherwise be dead can now live long and relatively normal lives. Illich is correct when he implies that those who develop diabetes at a young age suffer more in total than they did when they died early. But perhaps he should ask some young diabetics what they think of that.

Almost everyone recognizes that progress in the cancer field has been disappointing and would not quarrel unduly with Illich's claim that most modern treatment makes little difference to the outcome. But among the confusion and despair there are real signs of hope. Progress in charting environmental causes of cancer lends credence to the concept that as with the infectious diseases, with appropriate changes in the environment, many cancers will disappear. In the area of therapy there have been undeniable advances with chorion carcinoma, with Hodgkin's disease and with some leukaemias. These straws in the wind suggest that in principle the problem of preventing premature death from cancer is soluble.

For doctors not to recognize that their failure in the area of myocardial infarction is near total would be foolish. But for Illich to deny that the very impressive precention of strokes in known hypertensives as a result of medical treatment is a major advance is equally foolish. A stroke is one of the most devastating of all disasters to health. It often cripples without killing, converting active, energetic people into helpless hulks. To be able to prevent such a horror must surely be considered a medical advance. Similarly the surgical treatment of heart disease has its damaging and ridiculously exotic moments. But it undoubtedly leads to dramatically favourable results in an important group of patients.

Doctor-inflicted injuries

Illich gives a powerful description of the damage that doctors do to patients. Patients are made ill, mentally or physically, by the drugs which they swallow: they are subjected to unnecessary operations in a usually subconscious but occasionally conscious drive for surgical income: they are treated for diseases they do not have: they are subjected to diagnostic tests which may satisfy the doctor's scientific curiosity and may provide defence against accusations by other medical experts in a malpractice suit but which contribute nothing to the patient's well-being.

All these charges are partly true. What is uncertain is the extent of the damage caused and the amount of it which people of common sense would consider justifiable. In a society like the United States the legal system encourages lawyers to persuade patients to sue for damages by promising to waive any fee if the suit is unsuccessful but by claiming a large percentage of any award made. In this situation the majority of observers agrees that many of the suits filed are trivial and unreasonable. Yet even in the U.S.A. there were only about 15,000 malpractice suits per year in the early 1970's. If 25% of the population consult a doctor in one year this suggests a claim rate of about 1 in 3-4,000 doctor patient contacts. This hardly suggests a major epidemic of medical errors. In Britain and Canada where more realistic legal arrangements reduce suits to those which are likely to have a reasonable chance of success, the claims are a fraction of those in the United States. This suggests that legally-verifiable malpractice is at a level which is almost irreducibly low.

However, as Illich points out, malpractice suits can be successful only if a patient is considered to have been treated erroneously according to the accepted medical standards of the day. What may be more serious is the amount of damage done by treatment which medical experts consider acceptable. Neither Illich nor I has the evidence which would allow a reasoned statement on this point.

It is important to note that many of the side effects of treatment which can easily be attributed to the debit side by a polemicist are known and calculated risks taken by doctors often in consultation with their patients. Many forms of treatment which aim to alleviate or cure disease have inevitable side effects which cannot be dissociated from the therapeutic ones. Most surgery leaves patients at last temporarily much more ill than they would have been without surgery but that is hardly an argument against removing an inflamed appendix or an operable cancer or against repairing a hole in a child's heart. Many drugs make patients feel less well than they would otherwise be but that is not an argument for not treating a serious infection or a malignant growth which left untreated would make the patient considerably sicker than the treatment. Most patients understand these matters reasonably well. It is somewhat surprising to find Illich protesting so strongly since later in the book he makes it clear that he regards pain and distress as beneficial experiences.

Unfortunately it is probably true, as Illich says, that in the progression from a family practice to the research division of a university one becomes more and more likely to receive a treatment or, worse, be subjected to a diagnostic procedure which has consequences at least as serious as the disease. What he does not make clear is that this is because in the course of this progression patients approach areas where doctors are more and more aware that they do not have the right answers. There can be no doubt that the damage should be reduced but there can equally be no doubt that it is from this arena of struggle and uncertainty that the simple, safe, and effective procedures for use by future generations will emerge. The ethics of what happens in this arena are by no means clearly defined. There is undoubtedly a tendency on the part of some research-oriented doctors to subordinate the needs of the individual patient under their care to the supposed good of future generations of patients or even to the research prestige of the specialist units concerned. But this is a topic of very active debate and no one can say that the medical profession is currently ignoring it.

Defenceless patients

Illich summarizes his thesis by claiming that medicine is damaging individuals and society on three levels.

1. Clinical iatrogenesis consists of the damage done to individual patients by either wrong treatment, which would be susceptible to malpractice claims, or by the currently accepted correct treatment which would not. This is the main topic dealt with in the present chapter.

2. Social iatrogenesis consists of the damage done to society by medical practice which preserves defectives and which creates a demand for medical involvement in many areas of life where common sense and ordinary compassion would suggest that such involvement is at best unnecessary and at worst does great damage to human independence and dignity. This is dealt with in detail in the following three chapters. A point which Illich does not expand upon later is that our current morbid society 'industrially preserves its defectives'. I wish Illich had gone into more detail on this because I am not sure precisely what he means and I suspect that more information might have been revealing.

3. Structural iatrogenesis follows on from social iatrogenesis and is not always distinguished from it by crystal clear reasoning. What Illich seems to mean is a terminal state of individual and social dependence on medical care systems. This leads to a helpless feeling of individual uselessness, a failure to cope adequately with pain, disease and death and a requirement for medical processing through every stage of life. In this final state of nemesis, responses to pain, disease and suffering which previous generations would have regarded as healthy and normal are lost or considered pointless. In a 1984-like world all human life is placed in the hands of the medical profession.

Finally Illich makes one of the most crucial points of his whole thesis. He claims that there is no possibility of the medical profession reforming itself. He suggests that all medically devised measures which aim to protect the patient demand more medicine, not less. Even when such measures succeed in reducing clinical iatrogenesis (which they frequently fail to do) they increase social and structural iatrogenesis. In all the comments and reviews of Illich's work which I have seen, I have found no serious attempt to answer this point, the claim that just as the leopard cannot change his spots so the medical profession cannot reform itself. This is a disturbing omission. Even if Illich has exaggerated his case, there can be no doubt that medicine faces major problems. These problems are serious even if they are capable of correction by good medicine and by internal reform. If the problems are not amenable to such correction then one can only agree with Illich that the prospect is sickening in every sense of the word.

Radical change is required but I am still hopeful that medicine itself can initiate that change. This theme is developed in my final chapter. Even though I am not certain of being right, I am unequivocally certain that Illich's major proposal is wrong. To return medical care 'to the people' by removing controls and allowing lay individuals to supply and to accept medical care freely would lead to total disaster.

Hubris in classical literature was the human desire to acquire the attributes of the gods and to become involved in areas which are the prerogatives of the gods. Nemesis was the personification of divine resentment at this insolence on the part of man. The theft of fire from heaven by Prometheus and his subsequent eternal punishment was the archetypal story illustrating hubris and its inevitable consequence. As Illich says 'nemesis is the inevitable punishment of inhuman attempts to be a hero rather than a human being'. Illich believes that medicine has tried to be heroic, that it has thus lost its human attributes, and that in consequence it has brought down a terrible nemesis not only upon itself but upon society as a whole. My viewpoint is quite different. I can accept that Illich's description of the present situation is not totally out of touch with reality. I cannot begin to accept his account of the origins of the situation. Our current problems are consequences of the accumulating weight of small decisions made by small men and women with small concerns. Such people have been totally unaware of the huge consequences of what they have been doing. The image which best fits is not of a phalanx of Promethean heroes setting out to conquer the world: it is one of an army of peasants who by their small and immediate day-to-day concerns seriously damage the potential of a whole land. The medical profession has made great decisions without realising it. As was said of Britain, medicine has acquired its empire almost in a fit of absentmindedness. Having acquired it, it has no idea what to do with it.

I think that most people would agree that if there is a god and if he is concerned for humanity, he has enough respect for human independence not to interfere in such a matter as the organisation of medical care. If god does not exist, there can obviously be no question of his regarding medical care as his prerogative. Yet the decisions which face us in the medical field are undoubtedly ones which in a classical society would be considered the divine prerogative. We may not like the situation but we have no alternative to making heroic decisions. My thesis is that we have been unaware of this and have been ignorant of the great consequences of our apparently small decisions. Medicine has suffered not from too much hubris but from too little. Medicine must become aware that it is making decisions which the ancients might feel required divine intervention: it must make heroic decisions about its future in the full realisation of the impact these decisions will have. More hubris, not less, is required.

3 The Medicalization of Life

In this chapter Illich documents the way in which society is becoming increasingly dominated by medical considerations. In the 1940's forward-looking planners, especially in Britain were thinking about the development of health care systems open to all. It was frequently assumed that once such a system was freely available, and the existing burden of disease in society had been eliminated as a result of the newly acquired access to early medical care on the part of the poor, then the need for medical care, while not disappearing, would be substantially reduced. For three quite separate reasons this hope has not been fulfilled. Illich claims that instead of withering away, the medical care system has increasingly come to dominate society.

1. The illnesses which kill people prematurely tend to be short and sharp. When these diseases are almost eliminated, partly as a result of generally increasing standards of nutrition and sanitation, and partly as a result of effective medical treatment, then individuals do not become immortal gods free of all bodily ailments. Instead, the longer they live, the more they become afflicted with a range of chronic ailments. They therefore *want* more care for longer periods although as Illich points out the question as to whether they *need* more care is debatable.

2. Rapidly developing medical technology has succeeded in maintaining alive many infants who would previously have died and in beginning to tackle previously untreatable problems such as renal failure. It is interesting to note that when it suits the argument Illich is prepared to admit that medical care can sometimes be effective. But Illich's point is that in any terms the cost of such advances is huge and if we continue to devise 'successful' but extremely expensive ways of keeping people with severe health problems alive, the inevitable end result will be that the medical care system will become a Moloch, demanding more and more investment.

3. Most important of all, an attitude has been created in society which leads to a demand for medical care for an almost infinite range of problems. In only a small proportion of the situations for which it is demanded can medical care make an important contribution. The remainder consist of minor ailments for which in any sane society self care should be effective and of major ones in which medicine, despite its impressive

technological accoutrements, can do little to prolong survival or to improve the quality of life. Illich quotes a U.S. Department of Health official as saying that 80% of all funds channelled through his Department provide no demonstrable benefit to health. No proof is given and proof would be almost impossible to obtain. However, I have no doubt that whether the correct figure is 40% or 80% a large proportion of medical expenditure does no good whatsoever.

Illich believes that on balance, even in strictly clinical terms, more people are damaged by the health care system than are helped by it. This may or may not be true but no independent observer who reads the source material quoted by Illich can doubt that many people are damaged, although the damage may often be relatively trivial. The situations in which medical care genuinely saves lives and alleviates suffering represent only a proportion of medical expenditure. Much expenditure either makes no contribution, or at worst does serious damage or at best provides fulfilment for an abnormal emotional demand for health care, a demand which Illich believes should not be there at all. Illich claims that the health care system continually creates new demands and is in the position of the drug pusher who creates addiction in order to be able profitably to fulfil his needs.

Illich suggests that the situation is approaching a crisis point. Society will suddenly realise that the health care system is a fraud. Because health care has up to now enjoyed such high prestige, this crisis will then destroy not only the health care system but many other parts of the society as well. The only factor preventing this disaster – or triumph depending on one's point of view – is the ignorance of the public concerning the incompetence of doctors and the damaging effects of health care. Illich sees it as his mission to present clear concepts which will generate sufficiently powerful dissatisfaction to destroy the system as it exists. However, he admits that the emotional currents which he is creating may be used in one of two ways. On the one hand, health professionals will claim that the remedy is more investment in the medical care system, more and more research and more and more medical power. On the other hand, if the revulsion against medicine is sufficiently intense then the whole system will be discredited and dismantled. Illich believes that the second reaction is inevitable if only the public could be exposed to a statement in simple terms of what the health care system has already done. It is Illich's mission to provide such a statement so that populations may acquire the courage to recover their power for self cure.

Yet in the final paragraph of this section Illich makes an important point. He notes that the evidence he uses is not secret or difficult to come by. (This again is an interesting contrast to his claim in the first

20

chapter that the information is well repressed.) It is to be found in conventional medical journals and often in the most prestigious of them, such as the *New England Journal of Medicine* and the *Lancet*. This means that in a manner characteristic of no other profession at least some doctors are both aware of and passionately concerned about what is happening. Illich's belief is that the situation is hopeless and totally beyond reform by the profession itself. The sources of much of his evidence indicate that the situation may not be quite so gloomy and that much can yet be done. This theme will be developed in later chapters.

Dependence on care

Illich documents the changes in the cost of medical care during the past decades. And one has to admit that no matter how one looks at them only a word such as vast is appropriate to describe them. Illich is particularly concerned with the U.S.A., partly because of his North American experience, partly because of the amount of material available and partly because that country represents the ultimate offering – or threat – of Western medicine. In the last thirty years, the rate of rise of expenditure on hospital and other medical services has outstripped by four to six fold the average rises in expenditure on other items in the community. Most of the money spent has not gone to enrich doctors, even though they have certainly taken their share. I find it interesting that Illich has made so little of the issue of the wealth of doctors. He could have had a field day with it and it is evidence that he is not simply and blindly anti-doctor that he has been restrained on this issue. I think that it is a much more important issue than Illich recognizes. The extreme wealth of many North American doctors must be a matter of concern to the medical profession. When a medical degree becomes a passport not only to a lifetime of secure and fulfilling work but to virtually certain wealth, when a profession is so blind and so concerned with its immediate peers that it does not recognize how wealthy it is by almost any standards, there must be grave concern. Until very recently laymen have complained very little about the wealth of doctors. But voices are now beginning to be heard and the politics of envy seem to me more likely to generate an effective anti-medicine backlash than in any possible public recognition of medicine's inadequacies.

Although the United States offers the most spectacular examples of the increasing burden to the community of rising medical costs, Illich makes it clear that the fundamental phenomenon is near universal. The Northern European democracies, the Soviet Union, Eastern Europe and the developing countries have all experienced much the same sort of inflation of medical expenditure and medical influence. China temporarily and Tanzania perhaps more permanently may be exceptions to the overall pattern. Even in China Illich suspects that a highly technological system of medical care is being built up. The experience of a member of an American Medical Association delegation who recently suffered a heart attack while on a visit to China would support this. To the obvious astonishment of his colleagues the stricken man received highly sophisticated treatment virtually identical to that which he would have received at home. And he survived to tell the tale.

The increasing power of the medical profession as a whole is logically, though perhaps to some paradoxically, paralleled by a decline in the influence of all but a few individuals in the profession. This increasing power is not confined to any one political system. It tends to occur whenever individuals group together to form any society much larger than a village, irrespective of the political bias of that society. Throughout the world the supposed power and effectiveness of Western medicine is recognized. The unit costs of delivering Western style medical care are similar in all parts of the world yet national incomes per capita vary dramatically from country to country. Because of this Illich emphasises how inevitably inequitable the medical care system must be in all but a handful of nations. In poor countries only the very rich or those who are in some other way privileged, as are civil servants in Mexico, can have adequate access to the system. Again Illich seems to be arguing in a way different from that in other chapters. Elsewhere he claims that access to the medical system does damage. It is therefore presumably highly desirable to exclude as many people as possible from contact with medicine. I suppose he really means that the inequity lies in the actual distribution of the expenditure and not in the results of that distribution.

Again and again Illich returns to hammer home his point that while the ineffectiveness and huge cost of medical care are major issues, they are dwarfed in importance by the damaging effects which an increasingly dominant medical care system has on individuals and on their attitudes to themselves. 'More health damages are caused by the belief of people that they cannot cope with their illnesses without modern medicines than by doctors who foist their ministrations on patients.'

Illich clearly believes that there was a golden age when all people were sturdily independent of any dependence on any system for looking after the sick. He also believes that this healthy attitude has been destroyed by modern medicine. It is my belief that Illich is here putting the cart before the horse. I can find little or no evidence that most people have ever in any period of history believed that they themselves can handle their diseases. They have always looked outside themselves in seeking to cope with illness. They have turned to a priest, to a medicine man or to a patent medicine manufacturer. Quite reasonably, most people have difficulty in responding satisfactorily to their illnesses. For example, in a letter written to his brother Theo in April, 1881, Vincent Van Gogh wrote, 'The day after you left I stayed in bed, however, and had a long talk with Doctor Van Gent, a clever and practical man; not because I thought this insignificant malaise worthwhile, but rather because in general, either well or unwell, I like to talk with a doctor now and then in order to know that everything is right.'.

There have always been groups who have profited in terms of influence, or cash, or both, by catering to this inability to cope. For thousands of years only one factor has limited the influence of such people. That factor has not been the sturdy independence of individual human beings but the obvious failures of those who have claimed to know.

The yearning for real help in distress is no weaker than it has always been. The difference now is that there are quite unequivocal examples of the efficacy of Western medicine. Illich is right to draw attention to areas where modern medicine has failed but he condemns himself as unrealistic if he does not realise that the certainly limited but equally certainly very real power of medicine is obvious to everyone. This seems to me to be the secret of the influence modern medicine has over men's minds. It has genuinely begun to fulfil one of the most deeply felt of all human needs. What it must learn to do is to control itself so that if becomes involved only in those areas where its effectiveness is genuine. It must not use its limited power, whether by accident or design, to expand its influence over much wider fields.

Dependence on drugs

Illich points out that doctors themselves are not needed to sponsor dependence on modern ideas in medicine. In the absence of doctors over-enthusiastic drug marketing does the job almost equally well. In most rich countries there is close control over what medicines can be sold freely. Most of those which can readily do harm are restricted to use under medical supervision. In many poor countries, in contrast, potent drugs some of which are highly dangerous are freely available for purchase by anyone. These drug packages carry either highly technical instructions which could not be understood by a layman or simply a statement that they must be used under medical supervision. Either form of instruction is obviously nonsense in countries where, particularly in rural areas, there are few qualified personnel at any level.

I agree with Illich's analysis so far. As I know from my own personal experience, the indiscriminate way medical drugs are used in some developing countries is appalling. In the absence of adequate numbers of personnel, a situation which in most places is likely to persist for some time, more self discipline on the part of drug companies and more government regulation seem to me to be required. But beyond this point Illich's argument becomes to me incoherent. He is obviously disturbed by the unsatisfactory situation in the developing countries. Yet equally obviously this situation, where the doctors have no power to control drug use and where drugs are relatively freely available to all, is one which elsewhere in *Medical Nemesis* Illich advocates strongly. Without as far as I can see any logical link he therefore makes the statement, 'As drugs are being made increasingly into tools legally and technically reserved to the doctor, people are more prone to damage themselves with these drugs with or without a prescription. The medicalization of a drug renders it in fact more dangerous. Chloromycetin is a good example: for a decade it was prescribed against typhoid, against which it is effective, and also for many other conditions against which it is not and as a result aplastic anaemia became quite common. At the same time the absence of a clear warning about the dangers of the drug led people to use it on their own even when other treatment would have been quite as effective. Thus doctors and patients collaborated in the breeding of drug resistant typhoid bacilli now spreading from Mexico to the rest of the world.'

I may be missing something obvious but I frankly do not understand Illich's train of thought. It is not clear to me how medicalization made chloromycetin (chloramphenicol) more dangerous. Contrary to what Illich implies, the drug is genuinely effective in a wide variety of infections in addition to typhoid. It was in North America and Britain where medicalization of drugs is near complete that chloramphenicol was recognized to be a cause of aplastic anaemia. This aplastic anaemia (a total failure of production of red blood cells) was certainly not 'quite common'. It affected about 1 in 40,000 of those who took chloramphenicol. If he had been talking about drugs or doctors saving lives Illich would certainly have said that such an incidence was insignificant. But because he is discussing damage caused by a drug it suddenly becomes important. As a result of the recognition of this problem, in the countries where drug use is highly medicalized chloramphenicol became effectively restricted to use in typhoid, a disease in which there are few adequate alternatives. Aplastic anaemia due to the drug was thus virtually eliminated in these countries. As Illich says it was in countries like Mexico where medicalization is ineffective that aplastic anaemia continued to occur. Also in Mexico typhoid bacilli became resistant to chloramphenicol because of their repeated exposure to it when used for other infections in which effective alternatives are available. This seems to me a classic example of a situation in which effective medicalization sharply reduced the problems of using a drug while ineffective medicalization created a dangerous situation. It really will not do for Illich to say that this is an example of medicalization rendering a drug more dangerous.

In an aside which is also apparently inconsistent Illich praises Allende's idea that the pharmacopeia should be restricted to only a few dozen items of proven value. This seems to me to be medicalization in the extreme and I do not see how it fits into Illich's thesis.

Illich then turns to examples of the over-consumption of prescription drugs in industrialized countries. He rightly points to overuse of tranquillizers and other psychotropic drugs as a key problem. He shows that acquisition of drug dependence under medical supervision outstrips ways of becoming dependent on illegal drugs. He effectively disposes of the argument that the massive overprescribing is a consequence of drug company pressures. There is a close correlation between per capita income and per capita consumption of tranquillizers in all countries of the world irrespective of whether the regime is communist or capitalist. This is interesting, especially since what Illich does not do is to identify the driving force behind the rising consumption. If it really were a consequence of the behavior of the doctors and the drug companies one would have thought that the trend would have been much more pronounced in capitalist countries than in communist ones. The pressures to make patients use drugs superficially seem much more potent in the former. The possibility must therefore be considered that the over-consumption is not a consequence of the profession forcing unwilling patients to consume more drugs. Instead it may be insistent patient demand for some relief from problems deemed too great to be borne unaided. There is no doubt that in countries where tranquillizers are available only under medical supervision doctors could in part control the demand if they choose to do so. Nevertheless my own impression is that doctors are not in a Galbraithian sense generating a need and then catering to it. Instead they are making a largely ineffective response to a need which has probably always existed and would continue to do so even in the absence of all health professionals.

Medicalization of the life span

Illich complains that doctors have increasingly intervened in people's lives at all stages. People now require prenatal and neonatal care, special consideration when they are children and therapy for the simple state of being in their climacteric or old. Throughout their lives people are made to follow special medical routines in special health-producing environments. The overpowering emphasis on health 'degrades the quality of the home, the school, the street and the market place'.

I confess to having very little patience with most of this section. Is Illich really saying that prenatal and perinatal care which have done so much to reduce maternal and infant mortality and trauma during birth are bad things? He would find few mothers to agree with him. Is he really saying that people are currently being successfully regimented into medically approved regimes for maintaining health? He should look around in the streets of any big city or talk to any health education authority about the near-total resistance to propaganda about smoking, obesity, exercise and alcohol. The truth is that while people who feel even a little unhealthy have become unduly dependent on the medical profession, those who feel reasonably healthy are extremely resistant to the attempted medicalization of their lives. Those who are concerned with the prevention as opposed to the treatment of disease are very much aware of the eternal truth of John Owen's 16th century verse:

God and the doctor we alike adore
But only when in danger, not before;
The danger o'er, both are alike requited,
God is forgotten, and the doctor slighted.

Illich then goes on to say that because modern medicine can be very effective in the relief of certain symptoms, such as pain, it is not necessarily beneficial for the health of the patient. This is obviously true for some diseases such as the uncomplicated common cold or influenza for which medical treatment can do almost nothing. It is not true when those relatively tricial infections become complicated by the development of pneumonia. Nor is it true in the other extraordinary examples which Illich gives, namely tropical diseases and rheumatism. Modern medicines are remarkably effective in a very wide range of tropical diseases. This represents a major triumph of which those in the industrialized West are too little aware. The ability to treat protozoal and parasitic diseases such as malaria and hookworm means that people who would otherwise be chronically debilitated now have the chance to live full and normal lives. In no sense are these the acute and self-limiting diseases which Illich rightly says probably deserve much less medical attention than they receive. In the case of rheumatism it is true that the underlying disease process cannot be treated, but techniques of symptomatic relief are now sufficiently good to allow some people who would otherwise be totally crippled to live relatively satisfying lives.

In this section only when Illich writes about old age does he made much sense to me. Medicine has contributed to the reduction in death rates among the young and middle aged but has done little for the life expectancy of those who reach 65. They, on average, live little longer than they did a hundred years ago. In some ways by more effective measures of symptom relief medicine has made old age a little more tolerable. In others it has made life less tolerable by subjecting old people to heroic surgical procedures and potent drugs and by officiously striving to keep alive those whose lives should come to a quiet and dignified end. The care of the aged is an area where modern medicine has obviously already gone wrong and where the situation could get much worse in the near future. But it has gone wrong because it has mindlessly applied the maximum fire power of its available technology without considering the personal needs of individual patients. Doctors have increasingly refused to make Promethean decisions about withholding treatment and the present situation is a consequence of a lack of courageous decision making rather than an excess. This is an area where careful thought may lead to the conclusion that less medical care rather than more may lead to an improvement in health.

Finally Illich draws attention to a major mid-twentieth century tragedy. In developing countries that readily available, invaluable resource, human milk, is being used less and less and is everywhere being replaced by industrially prepared bottle feeds. As a consequence of this massive switch in infant feeding practices, there is a great financial burden in families and babies are exposed early on to abnormal and possibly dangerous patterns of nutrition. Infants run an increased risk of acquiring many infections because of the impossibility of maintaining adequate bottle hygiene under unfavourable conditions and they fail to receive the protective factors present in human milk which might help them to resist these diseases. Illich is correct to emphasise this tragedy but to say that it is a product of medicalization seems to be untrue and unfair. In the context of medical measures such as immunisation which are obviously helpful but which are largely administered by non-medical personnel Illich refuses to give doctors any credit. Even if doctors were in favour of the switch to bottle feeding, since the administration of the information about infant feeding is almost completely out of the hands of doctors, it is inconsistent to blame doctors for what has happened. But the truth is that as far as I am aware the switch from breast to bottle is almost universally condemned and vigorously resisted by doctors. It has occurred as a consequence of highly successful promotion by the commercial food giants, falling on the fertile ground of a female population which increasingly does not want to be continually tied to an infant and which wants to make use of opportunities for employment. Far from being an example of medicalization, this is a prime illustration of the fact that people consistently reject medical advice which does not seem to be in the immediate interest of greater satisfaction irrespective of the long term consequences.

Medicalization of prevention

Illich here concentrates his fire on the screening of or checking up on people who feel well by the use of full clinical examinations and the administration of batteries of tests. The purpose of such screening is to detect disease at any early stage when it is still perhaps treatable and has not done major damage. Much of Illich's case is justified. The benefits of routine screening have certainly not been proven and there is little published evidence to suggest that such routine screening leads to any increase in life span in the population exposed to an illness or to any decrease in the rates of death from any disease. The possible exception to this is screening for cervical cancer in women but even there the experts are arguing about the interpretation of the results. In contrast to its supposed benefits, screening may do considerable harm. It may utilize valuable resources which could be better employed elsewhere. It subjects healthy people to a procedure which is worrying, no matter how well informed they may be. It subtly creates an atmosphere in which people feel that no matter what their subjective sensations may be they may be unhealthy unless they have been screened and pronounced well.

But as so often in *Medical Nemesis,* having made a basically good case, Illich largely nullifies the impact by being extreme. He criticizes cardiac catheterization, a procedure in which the precise nature of heart disease may frequently be defined by injecting material which is opaque to x-rays into the blood and then taking a series of radiographs as it flows through the heart and its vessels. But cardiac catheterization could never even remotely be considered a screening process. With rare exceptions it is performed only on people who are already obviously ill, with the aim of defining precisely the nature of that illness. Illich then makes further errors when he implies that the only reason for cardiac catheterization is cardiomyopathy which is one of the least common indications, and he goes on to say that 1 in 50 people subjected to cardiac catheterization are killed by the procedure. This is an extremely serious error in a book written for laymen who may have to undergo such a procedure themselves. In fact the death rates from cardiac catheterization are around 1 in 1000. Cardiac catheterization is a vital preliminary to cardiac surgery in order to enable the surgeon to know what he is doing. Most of the deaths occur in those who are already seriously ill and whose lives would be short and miserable without surgical intervention.

Having digressed in this rather silly way, Illich goes on to make another crucial and entirely valid point. This is that many of the diseases which can be picked up by screening techniques are resistant to treatment. The patient, so long as he feels well, is often better off being ignorant about his illness for as long as possible. It seems to me obvious that screening should be strictly confined to those diseases which:

1. have serious consequences;
2. do not normally reveal themselves by symptoms until irrevocable damage has occurred;
3. are easily tested for, using techniques which do no harm;
4. are not very rare since otherwise very large numbers of healthy people will be subjected at great expense to worrying and useless investigation;
5. are effectively treatable since it is criminal even to try to screen for a disease if medicine currently has no beneficial effect on either morbidity or mortality.

If these criteria are applied, it is apparent that most proposed medical screening procedures do not begin to meet them. Routine antenatal screening does seem to do so since all women are worried about the outcome of their pregnancy, since it does not harm and since it does seem to have beneficial effects. Screening all newborn infants for congenital hip dislocation is another worthwhile procedure. This is a common abnormality, readily detected without any equipment other than human hands, easily correctable if picked up at birth but causing much misery and perhaps permanent deformity if not recognized until later. Most screening for cancer, with the possible exception of cervical cancer, is of uncertain value, partly because with many of the cancers treatment is unsuccessful. Screening for risk factors for heart disease will do no good until we can demonstrate that changing the risk factor alters the likelihood of developing the disease. A statistical association between, say, high cholesterol levels and heart attacks certainly does not necessarily mean that lowering the cholesterol level will reduce the risk. It may do so but equally it may turn out to be as valuable as cutting off the sores in the treatment of smallpox. Screening for hypertension is approaching the stage of being worthwhile since drug treatment has dramatically improved in recent years and can successfully prevent the strokes, the chronic heart failure and the kidney failure but not as yet the heart attacks which seem to go with the disease.

Illich is basically right about over-enthusiastic attitudes to screening in general but wrong in applying a blanket condemnation to its use in all situations. Paradoxically to many, but entirely logically to me, as in many other areas of medicine, better science will lead to more and not less humane treatment of people. The scientific approach has been sorely lacking in this field but is essential if we are to be able to define carefully those screening techniques which genuinely do lead to better treatment with a reduction in morbidity and mortality from a particular disease. If the science is done properly at the beginning, if wildly exaggerated and enthusiastic and quite unfounded reports are not fed to the public at an early stage, then screening will not be done in situations where its benefits are absent or uncertain but will be confined to ones where it is genuinely helpful.

Medicalization of expectations

There are several ways of approaching the battle between man and the diseases which attempt to destroy him. First there is the attempt to treat by genuinely effective technical intervention using drugs, surgery or other procedures such as dialysis for renal failure. Second, there is the provision of an atmosphere, a ceremonial which has no technical effect but which encourages the patient to use his own resources to fight the disease. Third, there is the teaching of the patient to tolerate patiently those conditions which are thought to be incurable. Fourth, there is the education and encouragement of the community as a whole to accept and not to reject, to care for and not to ignore, those who are sick. Finally, there is the very rare occurrence of miraculous cures which seem to transcend all common sense.

Illich suggests that all five aspects of the battle have now been taken over by medicine and its allied professions. Initially most of these tasks were performed primarily by religious or semi-religious individuals or societies. Then until very recently medicine shared the tasks with those non-medical groups. Now medicine has almost completely taken over and with procedures like heart transplantation has for many invaded the realm of the miraculous.

This description of what has happened is relatively accurate. But again Illich seems to me to confuse cause and consequence. His thesis seems to be that the invasion by medicine has occurred as the result of a deliberate Galbraithian effort on the part of the profession and that society is an ignorant and unwilling victim of medical imperialism. To me the order of events seems precisely the reverse. While the success of medicine are much more limited in scope than many lay people believe, they are nevertheless real. They are much more real than the successes of achieved by anything else in the fight against disease. No one follows the miracle worker who *never* performs miracles. The influence of medicine has invaded huge areas previously dominated by religion and by charity because it has achieved unequivocal, objectively verifiable and consistent results in certain areas. The invasion has been a liberation and has been welcomed with open arms. If the liberators do not achieve all that they promise, if sometimes the liberation has unfortunate consequences, that was ever the case and is accepted philosophically because no matter how disillusioning the reality, it is still better than the bondage which went before.

This confusion between cause and consequence again leads Illich to use contorted logic. For example, he writes 'The impact of symbols, myths and rituals on health levels is distinct from the effect of the same procedures in merely technical terms. An unnecessary or damaging shot of penicillin can still have a powerful placebo effect. As drugs became more effective, their symbolic side effects have become overwhelmingly health denying. In other words, the traditional white magic which supported the patient's own efforts has today turned black. Instead of mobilizing the patient's self healing powers, modern medical magic turns the patient into a limp and mystified voyeur'.

This is arrant nonsense. The first two sentences are unexceptionable but the rest is foolishness. What Illich seems to be saying is: 1. The success of treatment depends partly on its technical effectiveness and partly on the patient's determination to help himself and his belief in that effectiveness. 2. As therapy becomes highly effective (and here Illich is admitting subconsciously what he repeatedly denies elsewhere, namely that therapy is effective), because the patient believes in it completely, he ceases to have any interest in helping himself. 3. The effectiveness of therapy thus deprives him of a determination and independence of spirit which is a vital part of his humanity.

Some patients taken from tribal cultures and deposited in a modern hospital may certainly behave as though they had lost all interest in helping themselves. In Africa and Asia I have seen something like this happen. However my interpretation is that the 'limp and mystified voyeurism' is primarily a consequence not of excessive faith in the technical effectiveness of medicine but of a complete lack of faith in and understanding of a totally alien culture.

In my own experience of hospital wards in Britain, patients from societies which are already industrialised react to modern medicine in a very different way. They have an exceedingly healthy scepticism which results among other things in a widespread failure to self-administer prescribed treatments. They do believe that certain treatments can be effective but have grave doubts about others. Belief in the technical effectiveness of a treatment consistently increases rather than diminishes a determination to assist the treatment by self effort. Inevitably in every hospital there are willy wet legs who passively give themselves up to the doctors and nurses. But they form a group which would give up under any system and in any circumstances. They are certainly 'limp and mystified voyeurs', not only of medicine but of all life and it is grossly misleading to suggest that their behaviour is a consequence of medical intervention.

Illich uses as an example of the public's new dependence on medical miracles the astonishing South American tour of Dr. Christian Barnard who twice on the same day was able to fill the football stadiums in several major cities. Again my interpretation is different. This does not indicate to me an imperialist medical profession consistently striving to create a demand for miracles and then cynically and coldly fulfilling it. Instead it reveals a near insatiable demand which is already there which the medical profession, usually reluctantly and somewhat incompetently but occasionally boldly and with panache, has responded to. But no one should underestimate the disapproval within the profession for those mavericks who are somewhat too enthusiastic in their efforts to please the circus. Dr. Barnard's tour offers a prime example of what could happen to a susceptible public if all controls on the profession and on public access to medicines and techniques were thrown overboard.

Illich points out that the medical profession, or at least some of the more enterprising members of it, has used the public demand for miracles to persuade those who finance health facilities, whether public or private, to pay for high technology systems for the management of those with renal failure and for the care of those who have had operations, who have had heart attacks or who are terminally ill. There is some truth in his accusation but again the case is spoilt by indiscriminate exaggeration. Most would agree that in some modern institutions the techniques used to 'care' for the terminally ill have passed all bounds of sense. The value of coronary care units is debatable. There is unequivocal evidence that such units save the lives of some of those whose hearts stop or develop certain types of irregularity while in the unit. On the other hand there is some evidence that the stress of being moved to such a unit and cared for in it may itself initiate some of the disturbances. There is as yet no solid evidence that the net balance is in favour of being cared for in such a place. Yet in spite of this a high technology coronary care unit which gobbles up both capital and recurrent expenditure has become an indispensable status symbol without which no institution deserves the name of hospital. Far from being an instance of the mess that science can make, it is a prime example of a lack of a rigorous scientific approach leading to inhumanity and waste.

In contrast, there can be no doubt about the value of intensive post-operative care in terms of the comfort, the survival and the rapid recovery of those who have had surgery. Coronary care units became so fashionable in part because the value of post-operative care was so unequivocal. It was not realised that what was valid in one situation might not be so in another.

Illich reserves his most vicious rhetoric for the treatment by dialysis of patients with kidney failure. 'Consultants sanctimoniously select one in every five of those Englishmen who are afflicted with kidney failure and condition him to desire the scarce privilege of dying in protracted torture on dialysis. Much time and effort during the treatment is used in the prevention of suicide in the first and sometimes the second year that the artificial kidney may add to the lives of the patients.' The heavy sarcasm caricatures the true situation. Twenty years ago a diagnosis of bilateral renal failure almost invariably meant a rapid downhill course and a death within weeks or months at most. Many of the victims were young. Often they had small families. Their premature death was tragic in the fullest sense of that over-used word. Then first dialysis and later renal transplantation were developed as partial answers to the problem. The costs to society in financial terms and the strains on the patient in any terms were formidable. As Illich indicates some patients could not cope and attempted suicide. Selection of patients for dialysis had to be carried out partly because nowhere are there resources available to treat everyone with renal failure in this way and partly because many patients are psychologically unable to cope with the strain. On the other hand, some cope magnificently and their lives can be extended by several and perhaps many productive years. And for a man or woman with a young family even five years is of inestimable value. It can make the difference between the destruction of a family with young children and the survival of the mother or father to an age where the children are independent or nearly so. Should doctors really refuse to do anything about any patients with renal failure just because some cannot cope? Should they refuse the Promethean hubris of attempting to make a reasonable decision as to which patients should be treated and simply duck the issue by plucking names out of a hat? Or should they painfully, slowly and courageously work to ensure that those who do not want to be treated are allowed to die while those who desperately want to live, even at high cost, are enabled to do so? None of the people I have known involved in this is in the least sanctimonious. All have been humbly aware of the magnitude of the task, all have been unhappy about the procedures involved yet all have felt the effort worthwhile. To sneer can help no one.

Patient majorities

The chapter concludes with an encapsulated description of what Illich sees as the current situation. He claims that the medical profession is defining increasingly narrowly what it understands by a healthy normal person who requires no medical attention whatsoever. People who do not fall within these narrow limits are then classified as deviants of one sort or another. They therefore become patients under the tutelage of the profession. Only a small proportion of this group is genuinely ill by the standards of a previous generation. Others are being treated for trivial conditions or are not clearly ill at all but are being encouraged to bring one of their bodily characteristics which has strayed back into the realm of what is considered normal. Illich suggests that so many people are now classified as medically deviant that they have actually become a majority of the population in Western industrialized societies. Society is therefore dominated by this interaction between its members and the medical profession.

It is clear what Illich is driving at. A few doctors go to ridiculous and fanatical extremes to force their patients into the sort of narrow strait jacket which Illich describes. Worthy public spirited bodies tell people what is best for them so that, for example, seven of every ten advertisements to be seen in the buses of the city of Montreal relate to health matters. But fortunately while a few are believers most people, to the despair of health education propagandists, steadfastly refuse to take any notice. Illich's description is certainly a possible scenario for some time in the future if the trends which he has noted are not halted. As an account of what is now happening, it is yet another example of Illich's exaggeration.

4 Medicalization as a By-product of an Over-Industrialized Society

In this short chapter Illich sets what he believes about *Medical Nemesis* in the context of his thought as a whole. In all his books Illich has consistently contrasted what he calls the autonomous things which people do for themselves with the industrialized things which are done for people by modern society. Most economists and other thinkers have regarded industrialization primarily in connection with the production of goods. Some have argued that the most realistic way to limit growth and so to protect the environment will prove to be a shift in industrial effort from the production of material goods to the production of services. Education, health and leisure are seen as the growth industries of the future. Illich argues, rightly in my view, that this shift in emphasis is likely to be just as damaging as, in the past, traditional industrial effort has proved to be and people's ability to do things for themselves may be destroyed.

In such a service-orientated society, many aspects of which are already present in current industrial nations, people are conditioned to expect to be taught rather than to learn themselves; to travel by private or public power-driven machines instead of walking or cycling; to use the radio, the television, the tape recorder or the record player for entertainment instead of reading, making music or providing other pastimes for themselves; to expect all health care to be provided from outside instead of relying on maintenance of their own health by simple common sense measures.

It does not require long or profound thought in order to see that the thrust of Illich's argument is essentially correct. But in two important respects his understanding of what is happening seems to be wrong. First he underestimates the resistance of a minority who even in the most industrialised and packaged of societies insist on walking, on reading, on educating and entertaining themselves and on maintaining their own bodies in a healthy state with as little medical intervention as possible. No matter how totalitarian the state, this minority exists and within it are always to be found the seeds of downfall of the most all-pervading systems.

Secondly Illich overestimates the desire of the great majority of people to return to a more autonomous mode of existence which is usually classified by them not only as more autonomous but also as more primitive. He overestimates the satisfaction which most people who are to some extent autonomous not by choice but by force of circumstances find in that autonomy. Sturdily independent individuals, as Illich obviously is and as most educated people like to think they are, tend to imagine that everyone else feels (or at least should feel) the same way about what is a desirable pattern of existence. The majority of people do not feel that way.

The success of Western consumer products and services throughout the world, both in communist and developing countries, indicates that these things and concepts are inherently attractive to most people. There may be a need to work hard to sell one form of entertainment or one system of health care or education rather than another but there is little need to strive to sell the basic ideas. Most people do not seem to want to do things for themselves and given a free choice will opt not for autonomy and independence but for industrialization and dependence, provided that little effort is required. Those who provide more and more education or more and more medicine or more and more canned entertainment are not seen by the majority as conquering imperialists putting whole populations into slavery. Rather are they seen as liberators who are fighting to free people from all the drudgery that for those of limited intelligence and energy the autonomous mode of living implies.

If people really do want to live in an autonomous and independent way then, as Illich suggests, all we need to do is to remove all controls, to destroy the influence of all privileged professional bodies and people will then spontaneously seek autonomy in health, in education and leisure. On the other hand, if I am right the only way to restore even a moderate degree of autonomy to the majority is for those who have power and influence to display controlled hubris and to take Promethean decisions about matters which really should be left to the gods. But since the gods are manifestly not concerned, the only alternatives are hubris or mindless drift. One Eastern European country has tried the experiment, which would be virtually unthinkable in the West, of closing television transmission one night a week in order to stimulate the dying arts of conversation and home entertainment. That surely is a decision which could have been taken only by Prometheus and not by Everyman. It may be a pointer to the courageous sort of action which may be required if Illich's desirable society is to be achieved.

In another context in another age Goldsmith wrote:

Ill fares the land to hast'ning ills a prey;
Where wealth accumulates and men decay;

> *Princes and lords may flourish, or may fade;*
> *A breath can make them as a breath has made;*
> *But a bold peasantry, their country's pride,*
> *When once destroyed can never be supplied.*

By 'bold peasantry' I suspect that Goldsmith meant very much what Illich means by autonomous ordinary people. In the industrialised West that 'bold peasantry' has undoubtedly been destroyed by the seductive success of modern services. While 'never' may be too strong a word I think that Goldsmith rather than Illich is right in his assessment of the ease of restoration. I certainly do not believe, as Illich seems to do, that the abolition of all professional controls will lead to more autonomy on the part of ordinary people. My own guess is that it will lead to less. If any degree of autonomy is to be restored, those with influence and power are instead going to have to take some risky Promethean decisions.

Illich accepts (and as Carlyle might have said, 'Gad, he'd better') that some industrialization is inevitable. He even admits that it may be helpful to an autonomous way of life to produce certain items. The examples Illich uses are bicycles, books and strangely enough in view of the rest of *Medical Nemesis*, antibiotics. He is consistently curiously equivocal about antibiotics, either dismissing them as unimportant or condemning them as dangerous when it seems appropriate to the argument and praising them when their value is too obvious to be ignored. Nowhere is Illich prepared to admit the possibility that their obvious value may best be ensured by their strictly regulated professional use. However, this passage is interesting because it clearly indicates that Illich is by no means totally against industrial aids to medicine. It is only when the industrial aspects come to be completely dominant that the danger arises. It is unfortunate that this sane and balanced attitude is not maintained throughout the book.

Illich points out that there is a major practical problem in making a realistic assessment of the contribution to society of autonomous modes of living. Economists have devised crude but nevertheless moderately acceptable measures for estimating the magnitude of industrial output, whether in the form of goods or services. In contrast there are no even half reliable ways of assessing the importance of the autonomous mode. Since the total effectiveness of any effort to do anything in society depends on both autonomous and industrialized outputs, it is quite impossible to know whether that total effectiveness is increasing, decreasing or remaining static. Similarly since the autonomous mode is left completely out of the calculations, it is impossible to know who is benefiting and who is suffering from a particular change. In the case of medicine since we have no way of knowing how much independence of mind and spirit contributes to health, and since we have no way of measuring such independence, we cannot easily assess whether changes in medical care make a population healthier or not. Illich's implication is that almost all changes in medicine now reduce health, but the uncertainty is such that the opposite is certainly an arguable proposition. The industrialization of medicine so far has had little impact on most of the poor in the developing countries and so as yet they have been hardly damaged by it. It is certain underprivileged groups in the richest countries who are currently being most hurt. Illich takes the elderly in the United States as an example of this. As a result of constant interest in health matters on the part of newspapers, radio and television – which are undoubtedly only reflecting what the public wants – the elderly in North America have become aware of all the miracles of health care which seem to be technically possible. Yet there is no conceivable way in which sufficient resources could be pumped into the system to make such health miracles possible for all old people. As a result of life long exposure to services of many sorts, the ability of people to look after themselves has withered and the impact of this is greatest when with falling incomes in old age not all of the services can be paid for. Families have lost the ability and the will to look after their elderly and their only reaction to their relatives who may be infirm rather than ill is to put them in what is euphemistically called a home. Elderly people may therefore not even begin to cope (in a partially independent and emotionally satisfying way) with the very real problems which they face. Illich's nightmare is that the industrialization of medical and social services is going to proceed at an ever increasing pace. As it does so even younger people will be trained to believe that they are lacking in services which only the profession can provide. Eventually therefore the whole society will come to be in the dependent and frustrating position in which the elderly in the industrialized West now find themselves.

5 Futile Political Counter-measures

Illich contends that the state of the relationship between society and the medical profession is disastrous. One does not have to agree with him completely in order to see that there are at present very serious problems. The usual response to such problems is to attempt some type of political or semi-political reform. Illich discusses five types of reform measures which have been or could be proposed:

1. Regulation of the medical profession in order to ensure that it practises to the highest possible standards.
2. Public control of the delivery of health care so that the present inequalities of distribution observable in virtually every country are eliminated.
3. Public control over the internal organization of the profession in order to ensure that it behaves fully in the public interest.
4. Abolition of the exclusive recognition of and tax support for other approaches to medicine.
5. A switch from the idea that medicine should be orientated towards individuals to the one that it should be concerned with the health of populations and that it is the total environment which should be engineered in order to create a new medical system.

Illich rejects all these ideas as unrealistic. He contends that not only will each one fail to achieve its aims but will actually aggravate the situation. The attempt to reform will lead to further destruction of the individual's ability to care autonomously for his own health. Without necessarily agreeing with the more extreme statements he makes one can see that his view is probably valid. This will be brought out by discussing in detail the various proposed measures.

Consumer protection for addicts

The basic concept behind this approach is that the public performance of the medical profession should be carefully monitored and regulated. The aims are to ensure that only treatment measures which are genuinely effective are employed and that such genuinely effective measures should be administered in the safest possible way only to those patients who need them. Illich gives several reasons why this simply will not work.

First is the fact that laymen believe themselves incompetent to judge the quality of health care. They are quite happy to consider the merits and demerits of automobiles and household appliances. They feel able to make relatively realistic assessments about the costs and the benefits of proposed improvements and the relative balance between them. In contrast laymen do not regard themselves as competent to assess the relative values of various types of medical treatment nor to make any sensible estimates of the relative costs and benefits of proposed improvements.

It is true that laymen are at a severe disadvantage in attempting to assess the values of various aspects of medical treatment. But here as elsewhere Illich makes the incorrect assumption that the medical profession is a monolith with the will and the power to regulate all that its members may say and publish. As I have already pointed out by far the greater part of the ammunition which Illich uses to attack medicine comes from medical sources. Much has gone wrong in medicine but the profession has a great tradition of open discussion and free publication. There is never any shortage of lively-minded iconoclastic doctors who are willing to consider critically any situation in medicine. The fact that such doctors are in a minority and that they are often either ignored or vigorously opposed by the majority should not blind one to the facts that they exist and have an impressive record of winning in the end. As Ibsen wrote 'The majority is always wrong' and if the issues are discussed freely enough this will always come to be recognized. There will never be any difficulty in finding doctors able and willing to look critically at current treatment methods and systems of health delivery and to consider alternatives.

Second Illich emphasises the problems faced both by the lay consumer of medical care and by the professional health economist in assessing the relationship between the cost — in the widest sense of that word — and the benefits of any aspect of health care. The situation is unusual though by no means unique in areas where scientific and technical expertise is crucial. The assessors, whether professional economists or laymen, are in this situation dependent upon the suppliers of the goods and services to tell them whether the supply is satisfactory or not. Open public competition between individual doctors or between systems of treatment is vigorously discouraged and in most countries is punishable by expulsion from the profession. The economists' favourite laws of the market place are therefore not applicable and there cannot be any public decision in favour of one doctor or another. But Illich again misrepresents the situation in order to make his point strongly. He seems either to be unaware of or to underestimate gravely the vigour of the behind the scenes competition which goes on in medicine. There is sharp competition with few punches pulled in the struggle between alternative methods of treatment and health care delivery. Doctors are often independent-minded individuals and are not easily persuaded. The debates in professional journals and in meetings are in no sense controlled by any establishment. The lack of advertising by doctors and the lack of public competition for lay business which understandably give the outsider the idea that the profession is monolithic are in sharp contrast to the dramatic vigour of the internal disputes. Moreover, as Illich has discovered for himself, while the profession rarely sets out to inform the public about its internal disagreements there is no attempt to keep the information from public view. The issues are openly discussed in medical journals which can be purchased by anyone or consulted in any medical library. The level of informed criticism is such that genuinely ineffective treatments cannot now survive for very long if time is measured on a scale of decades. As I discuss in the last chapter, I fully accept that damaging treatments are often introduced far too widely at far too early a stage without proper evaluation. However, I believe that this is a problem which can be solved within the profession without recourse to external controls.

Illich makes the extraordinary claim that the medical profession is able to market its services to the public and that if necessary it will call on the police to force consumers to use its products. He is obviously thinking of the measures which are necessary in the control of epidemics and the detention of the violent. It would be naive to assert that the profession never misuses its potential association with the police but in Western democratic societies, serious incidents are rare enough to make the tone of Illich's statement strident and unconvincing.

In complete contrast the statement about the police is followed by a brilliantly eloquent attack on current approaches to the economics of health. This is a passage which should be studied carefully by anyone concerned in any way in this field. One passage is perhaps worth framing: 'The economics of health is a curious discipline, somewhat in the tradition of the theory of indulgences which flourished before Luther. You can count what the friar's collect, you can look at the temples they build, you can take part in the liturgies they indulge in but you can only guess what the traffic in amnesties for purgatory does to the soul after death. Models developed to account for the rising willingness of taxpayers to foot rising medical bills provide similar scholastic guesswork about the new world-spanning church of medicine.' Everyone knows the value of health but no one can yet adequately evaluate the role of medical expenditure in keeping people healthy.

Illich believes that reform of the health delivery system is impossible because ultimately such reform depends on advice given by doctors. Any representative committee of doctors or of doctors and laymen appointed to investigate the situation is likely to assume that the system may have its defects but is nevertheless basically satisfactory. No committee is going to come up with recommendations for executive action which involve more than a little tinkering with standards here and there. No committee is going to come up with a conclusion that the majority of doctors is wildly at fault in its delivery of health care. All such conventional techniques of reform are therefore doomed to failure. If anything they are likely to result not in a decrease in the medical regulation of individual welfare but in an increase. Illich's position is that 'control over the production side of the medical complex can work towards better health only if it leads to a very sizeable reduction in its total output rather than simply to technical improvements in the wares which are offered.' He may well be right both in saying this and in his unstated assumption that the medical profession will never recommend this. However as will be clear in the last chapter, I retain some faith in the profession's ability to take a hard look at itself and believe that it may yet surprise both itself and Illich by coming up with some radical new solutions.

Egalitarian access to torts

The approach of most radical critics of medicine is to assume that there are only minor defects in the technical aspects of medical care. The real problem is thought to be the serious maldistribution of medical care in almost all countries. For Illich, of course, this approach is naive. He believes that the medical care system is harmful anyway. If the system is to be open to all, in most countries it will have to be dramatically expanded. It will then have the opportunity to do even more damage. As he succinctly puts it in the heading to the section, what these radical critics are wanting is egalitarian access to torts. The poor would actually be harmed by easier access to 'quality' medical care.

Even if this view is correct it does not justify the gross maldistribution of resources and the expenditure of tax money on the privileged only. The education of a doctor takes vast sums of money and in poor countries this is out of all proportion to that spent on other forms of education. Yet in the end, with only rare exceptions, most such doctors spend their time treating the rich only, often abandoning government service for private practice. If the government tries to regulate the profession, the individual doctors tend to leave for North America or Western Europe constituting a substantial form of aid from the developing to the developed and making it difficult to justify the expenditure on their education. Unfortunately such governments are often not rational.

Illich discusses in some detail the example of Mexico where government employees at any level have totally free access to an outstanding health care system whose standards are as high as any in the world. Labourers and heads of government departments seem to receive genuinely equal treatment. Yet only 3 percent of the population is in government service whereas the scheme takes one-third of the national health budget. If care of a similar standard were to be extended to the whole population the Mexican medical budget would have to be increased more than ten fold, excluding any capital investment in buildings, equipment and the education of personnel. It could not be done.

As mentioned earlier Illich genuinely believes that if such an impossibility did come about then the poor would actually be harmed, not only in the sense of an erosion of their independence but in a technical clinical sense as well. In order to demonstrate this he uses the fact that the United States ranks 17th among the nations of the world in the infant mortality stakes in spite of its high medical expenditure. He points out that this cannot readily be accounted for by lack of finance since he provides documentation for the fact that surprisingly large sums are spent on medical care for the poor in the U.S.A. He therefore attributes at least part of the high infant mortality to 'collision with an over-equipped medical system'. This argument does not hold water. First Illich ignores the *quality* of medical care and makes no attempt to distinguish between that and the medical time and dollars spent. It seems to be agreed by doctors of broad international experience that while the best American medicine is the best or as good as the best in the world, the worst, which may be almost as expensive, is very bad indeed. Second Illich ignores the fact that although plenty of dollars are spent on medical care for the poor pregnant mother and her infant, more are spent on the rich. Infant mortality rates for the American rich are much better than for the poor yet if Illich is right the reverse should be true. Thirdly in the Northern European democracies where the standards of medical care are much more even and good quality medicine is genuinely available to all, differences between rich and poor in infant mortality are much smaller and overall infant mortalities are lower. Therefore it is very unlikely that the high U.S. infant mortality rates can be attributed to contact with a medical care system which is both expensive and of good quality. It is much more likely that the figures are a consequence of a combination of poor social conditions among the underprivileged and exposure to high cost but nevertheless poor quality medical care. Illich implies that he understands this when in a later paragraph he attributed the poor health of the American child to crowding, pollution, crime, discrimination and (my italics) *second rate contact with the health system.* 'Extra therapy *of the kind now offered* adds to the total negative impact which a poor environment has on the health of the poor. Less access to the present health system would, contrary to political rhetoric, benefit the poor.'

It is possible that this may be true of the United States but it is misleading to make the implied generalizations from the poor of that country to the poor of the rest of the world and from the health services offered to the American poor to those offered to the American rich and to those available to all in the Northern European democracies. There is no evidence that I know of that in these last countries the poor are clinically harmed by contact with the health care system.

Whether Illich is right or wrong about the effects of modern health care he is certainly correct when he says that access to up-to-date medicine has become a status symbol (although one suspects that it has been throughout history). Such access is as important to the lay public as are the technical results of treatment. As a consequence in a democratic society which genuinely reflects the public will, elected representatives will always tend to do what the profession wants. Most lay people feel that apart from doctor's salaries what the profession wants is likely to be in the public interest. I agree absolutely that this is one of the mainsprings of the power of medicine. But I cannot see how Illich fits this in with his concept that removal of all controls would lead to the public choosing a more autonomous way with less medicine rather than more. He is certainly right — and this is something which the shrewder members of the profession are beginning to understand — when he states that the most effective way for the profession to get more resources allocated to it is to combine advanced research on high technology medicine with a loud demand for equal access for all to this type of 'big medicine'. 'Public control of a growth orientated medical profession will reinforce its health denying expansion'. In truth only the profession itself is in a position to decide that the time has come to contract its services and that requires a degree of courage and of hubris which is Promethean indeed.

Public control over the medical mafia

Illich here discusses the consequences of public bodies attempting to regulate the internal organization of the medical profession. The two aspects with which he deals are the financial rewards of medicine and the overwhelming influence of doctors within the total health system.

In countries without some sort of government-controlled National Health Service — and even in some countries with one — doctors are frequently the most consistently rich members of society. Many feel strongly that in a profession which is supposed to be a vocation this should not be so. It is a point of view with which I have considerable sympathy. One would have thought that this might be something which

Illich would hammer with all the rhetoric at his command but surprisingly he lets the doctors off lightly. This indicates to me that contrary to what some members of the profession believe Illich is not crudely and simply anti-doctor. He contends that the wealth of the profession, although it may be offensive, does nothing to harm the public. This follows from his contention that all contact with the health care system is harmful. In the countries where the profession is richest the distribution of medical care is most uneven and the poor are to some extent protected against medical excesses.

Illich makes the nicely Machiavellian point that obvious public irritation over medical wealth is a useful check on the real power of the profession. If doctors really did become dedicated and worked long hours for low salaries there would be few limits to their public prestige and power. The rogues offer a most useful antidote and Illich is very much against doing anything to control them. 'Public control over the private enrichment of a few individuals could easily become a powerful device for legitimitizing an even more intense medicalization of life.' He is probably right but his approach is a tactic worthy of a Renaissance prince.

The power of doctors within the health care system, with the consequent reduction of other professionals to the status of second rate citizens, is another source of irritation. This has resulted in demands for a more elevated status for all types of health professionals ranging from nurses to social workers. Since the doctor's superior education has been thought to be a major source of his power, attempts are constantly being made to increase educational requirements for other professionals. This manoeuvre has been carried out very successfully without apparently increasing by one iota the ability of such professionals actually to perform their work. As a result the public is faced not only by the doctors but by a whole range of other professional groups, each determined to raise its status even further and to increase its share of the empire. The situation has parallels in the 19th century imperialist scramble for Africa. The end result of this internal competition is an inevitable expansion of the domination of the health professions as a whole.

Even within medicine itself, the proliferation of specialities tends to have a similar effect with each group competing for patients and with little coordination between them. Again this is more true of the United States than elsewhere. It points strongly to the need for a patient to have a primary relationship with one general practitioner who will help him or her to chart a sensible path through the medical unknown.

Tax support to all medical sects

The medical profession is no longer only a practical group of people who use their skills to attempt to help sick people. It has become a world-wide Church whose lofty aim is the 'salvation of mankind from shackles of illness, impairment and even the necessity of death'. It 'has come to play a role formerly reserved to the priesthood, using scientific principles as its theology and technicians as its acolytes'. Again Illich's description is not too far from the mark.

Illich seems to be antagonistic to the part which science plays in medicine. He feels that this increases the control which doctors have over patients and leads to attempts to regulate things which should not be regulated. D.H. Lawrence put it very succinctly:

> When I went to the scientific doctor
> I realised what lust there was in him to
> wreak his so-called science on me
> and reduce me to the level of a thing
> So I said: Good morning! and left him.

Illich, Lawrence and not a few doctors do not understand what science is all about. The thing they are attacking is not science but technology and a caricature of technology at that. But we must recognise that such a caricature of technology is indeed what some doctors understand by science and that the complaints of Lawrence and Illich are justified. As I shall demonstrate in the last chapter of the book, better true science would decrease rather than increase doctor control of patients. It is the invocation of science as a sort of cure-all saint's relic by doctors who themselves neither understand it nor believe it which causes most trouble.

At the moment in most countries, though not in all, the medical profession itself decides who shall be admitted to the priesthood. Eccentric practitioners of all types are refused recognition and therefore usually financial support from government sources. One form of radical criticism of medicine suggests that this monopoly position of orthodox medicine in relation to the public should be terminated and the medical church disestablished in the sense of having its connections with the state terminated. There are numerous religious precedents for such disestablishment. Such a measure would then open government financial support for all types of eccentric practitioners including homeopaths, Ayurveds, acupuncturists and witches.

Illich is not purely concerned with the impact of orthodox medicine on man. Because that is so powerful it is currently the most important. But what worries Illich is the total sum of the control of health matters by people who call themselves experts whether they are orthodox or not. He rightly argues that the subordination of a society by medicine would be made more emphatic by such a multiplicity of medical sects. With such a range to choose from most people will find some health care system which satisfies them and even greater numbers than before will resort to medical control of some sort instead of relying on themselves. This type of solution while undoubtedly decreasing the power of orthodox medicine would actually increase the total sum of the power of health professional groups. As Illich says medical care systems are currently limited by the irrational control over irrational systems exerted by doctors. This leads to less iatrogenesis and damage to society than would occur if either the orthodox system were rationalized or if the doors were thrown open to competing systems. Either remedy will only deepen the sickening effect of medicine and decrease the extent of the areas left open to self care.

I agree strongly with this analysis but as so often it seems to me that the arguments which Illich marshalls so potently effectively destroy his own proposed solutions.

Engineering for a plastic womb

The four categories of strategy for the reform of medicine so far considered in this chapter are all, like orthodox medicine itself, based on care for the individual no matter how inadequate and incompetent such care may be. The fifth strategy involves a quite different approach. Essentially it claims that man is unhealthy because the environment is unhealthy and that the only sensible approach to care for the individual is to create a total environment where illness is unlikely to occur. Diet must be supervised, pollution of all types must be controlled, education must be regulated. Everyone will then grow to be an optimally fed, physically and mentally healthy adult.

If limited by common sense and respect for individuality, there is nothing wrong with this approach. There is nothing wrong with searching for toxic agents in our food and environment and then trying to eliminate them. There is nothing wrong with trying to teach people simple health care. But Illich fears that such environmental engineering will not stop there. He suspects that the common sense distinction between health and ill health will be further distorted. More and more deviants will be labelled patients even though they are in no sense experiencing anything which anyone fifty years ago would have recognized as a disease. This approach may give a new legitimacy to 'total treatment' and the power and influence of the health professions will expand even further. The labelling of all sorts of social deviation first as crime and then as sickness will give new authority to the medico-political control of individuals 'in their own interest' and the invocation of scientific medicine will reduce the ability of individuals to resist totalitarian attitudes. The attempt in both the democracies and the communist countries to label implacable apponents of the government as sick — though at present much more obviously used in the Soviet Union than the West — indicate the ways in which medicine could be used as a tool for the further subjection of individuals. Again Illich exaggerates but it is all too easy to be overly complacent on this point. It is an area where eternal medico-legal controls over individual action, such as the prohibition on driving by epileptics, seem common sense. But the distinction between what is sensible and what is not is quantitative rather than qualitative. It is a situation where perfectly ordinary people may take things to ultimate logical conclusions and become fanatical. What is permissible and what is not must not be settled by committees sitting behind closed doors but by open and continuous debate with free participation by both laymen and professionals. Without such debate even men of good will may start acting in the interests of others and applying controls which are clear infringements of liberty.

In this chapter Illich therefore concludes that not one of the proposed strategies for reforming medicine will achieve its desired end. Some strategies will fail but even ones which apparently succeed will inevitably result in increased iatrogenesis. As I shall show later in the book Illich's own solution has precisely the same defect.

6 The Destruction of Medical Cultures

Up to this point while I have differed strongly from Illich with regard to details I have been in broad agreement with his overall assessment. I am in sympathy with his description of the situation, even if not with his understanding of the reasons for the state of affairs. But now I begin to deviate sharply from his analysis and I find myself less and less sympathetic to what he says. I have tried to deal with all points courteously and effectively but the reader who detects a subtle — or not-so-subtle — change in my fundamental attitude is not wrong.

Illich starts with an assumption which, so far as I am aware, is not formally proveable. Nevertheless I agree with the sentiments. 'The well-being of men and women increases with their ability to assume personal responsibility for pain (and) impairment (and it depends on) their attitude towards death'. He continues 'Man, modified by a particular place and companionship, simply does not exist. He has never existed in this condition nor could he ever survive in this way.' (Incidentally this explains why personal biographies are so important in understanding thought processes and why it might be helpful if Illich could let us have more details of his.) 'Culture, in other words, is the particular form that survival, coping and viability take in a given human group.' Health care is an essential part of this culture which cannot be logically separated from it. Man free of all cultural determinants does not exist. There is no such thing as either the natural man of classical anthropology, free of all cultural determinants, or the consensual man of modern anthropology consisting of the elements common to all cultures. Illich claims that both these views 'transform individual eccentricity and distinctiveness into deviation, impairment and sickness by insisting on the underlying, unchanging normative type of man as the formal object of scientific enquiry'. Illich says that 'to become human, the individuals of our species always needed to discover a particular programme by which to conduct themselves in their struggle with nature and neighbour. In this struggle they would often be on their own but the weapons and the rules and the style for the struggle were supplies by the culture in which they grew up. Each culture evolved and defined the way of being human or healthy in its unique way. Each group's code suits a given genetic make up, a given history, a given geography and the necessity of facing a set of other

48

cultures. Each group's code changes according to this total environment. Along with the culture, men evolved, each learning to keep alive in this common cocoon. Each culture not only provides instruction for tilling and fighting but also a set of rules with which the individual could come to terms with pain, impairment and death'.

Here Illich makes a fundamental error. The first five chapters of his book are entirely devoted to the importance of the individual and to the need for the individual to be able to care for himself in an autonomous way. Illich is vigorously opposed to anything which would reduce, that autonomy. Some of his most pungent criticisms are reserved for those who are trying to engineer an environment which is totally healthy. He rightly fears that such an environment, while providing complete security for those under its umbrella, would suppress as deviant and unhealthy most forms of individual expression.

Yet only a few pages later, Illich extols the virtues of traditional cultures which do precisely what he so strongly condemns. They provide in his own words, 'a common cocoon' which prescribes exactly what the individual should do in every situation. They offer a system of health care which cannot be distinguished from the culture as a whole. Why this, which a few pages earlier had been anathema, should now suddenly become acceptable because it is old rather than new is a mystery to me. The prime virtue of traditional systems of care is their concern for the total man and their insistence on providing rules for every eventuality so that if the individual keeps to these rules he can feel safe.

To use Illich's own classification of types of harm, in terms of clinical iatrogenesis traditional systems are disastrous. No one who has seen the victims of traditional care in a tribal society can avoid this conclusion. Traditional care has its rare successes: in many cases it does neither harm nor good clinically: but in many other cases its impact is appalling. Many individuals have had their lives completely ruined by it. Similarly in terms of social and structural iatrogenesis, the rigid traditional systems dominate both the individual and the society in which he lives. They generate the feeling that the individual can do little or nothing for himself because he is constantly in their grip of forces and powers beyond his control. Traditional cultures exhibit to the ultimate degree all the evils which Illich attributes to modern industrialised medicine and which in a complete volte-face he now finds so appealing. The variety of traditional cultures and therefore the variety of lives which man may lead must now obscure the fact that within any one such culture deviance by an individual is regarded with much greater hostility than it is in the modern industrial state. The fact that an individual in such a culture feels secure is not because of his autonomy but because of his complete dependence on a set of traditional rules. The success of traditional medicine does not lie in its clinical competence where disaster is a more likely outcome than success. Nor does it lie in the freedom and self-confident independence it gives to individuals. Traditional cultures can be successful because they instil the confidence that because of long human experience all answers to all questions are known. All one need do is follow the rules and one will be safe.

It is unacceptable for Illich to criticize modern medicine so vigorously and then, simply because they are traditional, to advocate systems which exemplify to near perfection all the things which Illich seems to be fighting so hard against. Personal responsibility for the welfare of oneself and others is an idea which has only recently achieved any substantial degree of acceptance among ordinary people. For perhaps two or three centuries it has flourished vigorously in a few Western European nations and their offshoots. It now seems almost everywhere to be in decline. Illich's complaints about modern medicine are really complaints about an impending return to a traditional type of health care, which because it is comfortable and apparently safe seems to be what most men require. Society and the experts will tell us what to do in every situation. What we should be doing is what Illich does relatively successfully in the first two parts of his book, not struggling to so return to a traditional cocoon, but fighting to conserve, to consolidate and to build on the gains we have already made.

Having praised the traditional approach, Illich condemns modern cosmopolitan medical civilization for denying 'the need for man's acceptance of pain, sickness and death. Medical civilization is planned and organized to kill pain, to eliminate sickness and to struggle against death. These are new goals, and goals which have never before been guidelines for social life. From being essential experiences with which each of us has to come to terms, pain, sickness and death are transformed by medical civilization into accidents for which people must seek medical treatment'.

This is nonsense. Modern medical culture certainly accepts the inevitability of death even though it struggles against it, sometimes nobly and successfully, sometimes unwisely and disastrously. Most traditional cultures have methods, either psychological or technical, for attempting to heal disease or to reduce its impact and to relieve pain. To say that these are new goals is ridiculous. But whereas in traditional society it was accepted that these goals would for the most part not be achieved and therefore that resignation was the only sensible answer, it is now widely believed — and correctly so — that most pain can be alleviated and that much sickness can be relieved. I fail to see why pain relief and the healing of disease should be so unequivocally damaging even if they were as Illich claims completely new goals never previously sought by man. At some times Illich's historical sense seems well developed but at others, as here, it is curiously weak. All traditional cultural customs and techniques for facing sickness and death must have been new at some time. It is naive to forget this just because the time at which they were new is lost in obscurity and is not the subject of written records. Man is man because he consistently sets new goals for himself. This is undoubtedly a stressful exercise but the fundamental psychological problems have been coped with in the past. In spite of the apparent dramatic increase in the rate of change, I am reasonably confident that man has a good chance of coping again with his new aims.

A point which Illich ignores is that in all traditional cultures the distribution of pain and sickness is hopelessly inequitable. If it is right that all should pass through the essential experiences of pain and sickness at a time when they can learn from them, then pain and sickness should be deliberately inflicted upon those who have temporarily escaped. The brutal initiation ceremonies among some peoples may be attempts to do this. On the other hand if it is right that even in traditional societies some people should live healthy lives, free of serious pain, then why is it wrong to attempt no matter how unsuccessfully, to extend these same privileges to all? I believe that the instinct of the great majority of mankind, that pain and sickness are evils which it is better to eliminate rather than to bear stoically or even masochistically, is absolutely right. There is nothing wrong with medicine's effort to relieve pain.

What is required is a common sense approach which enables decisions to be made as to when the efforts of medicine are damaging and when life giving in the broadest meaning of that expression. For me the controlled rage shown by the best doctors when confronted with impossible pain and incurable disease is one of the best aspects of medicine.

In the last paragraph of the chapter Illich sets out explicitly what he means by *Medical Nemesis*. This is such a crucial passage that it would be unfair and unwise to paraphrase it. 'The increasing attachment and allegiance to therapy affects the social character of a people. An idolatrous demand for manipulation comes to be identified with health care and replaces autonomous confidence in biological vigour, the wisdom of traditional rules and the compassion of neighbours. When dependence on the professional management of pain, sickness and death grows beyond a certain point, the healing power in sickness, patience in suffering and fortitude in the face of death must decline. These three regressions are symptoms of third level (structural) iatrogenesis: their combined outcome is Medical Nemesis.'

Illich greatly expands these themes in the following chapters and I shall reserve most of my comments until then. Here I should simply like to pose a few questions. Why should a demand for health care be idolatrous and what does Illich mean by this? What is the evidence that confidence in biological vigour is common among people not exposed to modern industrial medicine? Why should traditional rules be considered to be always wise? How reliable is the ccmpassion of neighbours especially in chronic and socially unacceptable illness? What is the healing power in sickness? Why should those who suffer be patient? Why should death be faced with fortitude in situations in which it is not inevitable?

Illich here begins to move far away from what Everyman understands and desires. Illich is creating a society for Promethean heroes. The emptiness of his argument is obscured only by the brilliance of the language in which it is expressed.

7 The Killing of Pain

For Illich pain is an experience of the profoundest religious and philosophical significance. Every human being should suffer it. Pain is a crucial factor in the development of human personality. To pain are ascribed innumerable virtues. 'Patience, forbearance, courage, resignation, self control, perseverance and meekness each express a different colouring of the responses with which pain sensations were accepted, transformed into the experience of suffering and endured. Duty, love, fascination, routines, prayer and compassion were just some of the means that enabled pain to be borne with dignity.'

Illich reacts strongly against the idea that pain is a concept which should be narrowly interpreted and which should be limited to those physical sensations which accompany damage to or destruction of a particular part of the body. It is essential that pain should include the emotional assessment of the meaning of pain for the individual. This caring about the wider implications of a sensation of pain is certainly something which many doctors are careless of. But for Illich the implications are extraordinarily wide. They include not only matters of relatively direct significance such as assessments of how long the pain is going to last, whether it is going to get better or worse, whether it means any serious illness or disability or whether it is going to end in death. Pain includes all the anguish of being human in an imperfect world and is an essential experience if we are fully to understand our porition on this earth. Pain is an indispensable mirror to delight and is a constant reminder to human beings — who might otherwise forget — that they are mortal and dependent upon one another. Pain is the experience which transforms children into adults and which gives people confidence in their ability to cope with 'triumph and disaster and to meet these two impostors just the same.'

In Illich's view pain must be accepted by individuals as an 'inevitable part of their conscious coping with reality'. The way to deal with pain is to see it in the context of a culture which 'confronts pain, deviance and death by interpreting them'. 'Culture makes pain tolerable by integrating it into a meaningful system.' 'Bodily pain, experienced as an intrinsic intimate and incommunicable disvalue, includes in our awareness the social situation in which those who suffer find themselves.'

53

Even Illich recognizes that most people see pain as an evil and at
some times require relief by drugs. His answer is to remove the relief
of pain from medical control and to make traditional pain-relieving
remedies — including opium — freely available to the public to use in
any way they will. Opium and alcohol are to be accepted as pain relievers because they have 'always been used'. Again Illich's historical
sense deserts him. At some time in pre-history, man for the first time
experienced the delights of alcohol and opium. Those were entirely new
experiences with which he had to learn to cope. I see no reason to
believe that man is any less able to cope today.

But for Illich the drug relief of pain is a side issue. The central factor
which enables man to cope with pain must be his experience of traditional culture. Culture 'allows individuals to deal with their own pain.
The act of suffering is shaped by culture into a question which can be
stated and shared. Culture provides the vehicle for expressing pain: the
sounds and gestures that communicate and relieve. It also supplies the
grammar to understand the pain as a challenge to be borne with dignity:
the need to behave in a certain fashion distracts attention from otherwise all-absorbing sensations. Finally, culture supplies the myth with
which to interpret pain: as Kismet to the Muslim, as Karma to the Hindu,
as a sanctifying backlash of sin to the Christian, to others vengeance,
punishment, the evil eye or simply a mystery.'

These ideas of Illich are scattered through the chapter. I have attempted
to bring them together in order to provide a coherent view of Illich's
concept of pain and its meaning. Also scattered through the chapter are
an account of the historical development of medical ideas about pain
and Illich's comments on the disastrous nature of current medical responses
to pain. I shall try to summarize these before presenting my own views
on Illich's ideas.

In Greek medicine pain was an important guide in diagnosis. It revealed
to the physician which harmony of the body was out of tune and had to
be recovered. Thus the relief of pain was not one of the primary aims
of medicine although it might occur as a secondary consequence of
successful therapy. This attitude permeated the Western tradition until
the 17th century claims Illich. 'Anaesthesia, as opposed to the solace of
prayer, wine or poppy was surprisingly absent from medical practice and
from popular expectations.' (Illich does not consider the possibility that
this attitude may have arisen from a belief that anaesthesia was simply
not possible.) For the few pain was sometimes an instrument of divine
punishment; for the Christian almost always so; for the neo-Platonist
the result of a deficiency in the celestial hierarchy; for the Manichee
the result of positive malpractice on the part of evil forces. In all Western

cultures pain was 'the bitter taste of cosmic evil', either a well-deserved divine curse, a manifestation of a flaw in the structure of the natural world or the expression of a diabolical will. For Illich this idea of the experience of the bitter taste of cosmic evil is at the core of any healthy attitude towards pain. Pain should not be relieved except by opium and alcohol which 'have always been used'. Pain should be handled by heroic defiance or stoic acceptance and welcomes as an opportunity for purification, penance and sacrifice. The relief of pain as an end in itself in traditional Western culture was unthinkable. Illich says this was because pain was regarded as a symptom of cosmic not individual distress, a sign of the corruption of nature of which man was a part and which could not be eliminated without eliminating man, an experience of the soul which was present throughout the body and indistinguishable from it. 'Pain was a non-mediated experience of lack or of evil. There could be no source of pain distinct from pain itself.'

It was Descartes who crystallized ideas which had been emerging over previous centuries. He made an unequivocal distinction between body and soul, thus making it possible for pain to be regarded as an experience of the body not necessarily intertwined with one of the soul. For Descartes — and this idea was rapidly developed by his successors — pain was simply a signal that some part of the body was in danger. This signal was transmitted to the soul which whenever possible took appropriate action to eliminate the danger and so to relieve the pain.

By the second half of the 19th century for Western medicine and science pain was simply a regulation of bodily function. It was subject to natural law, undeserving of any mystical respect, and did not require any metaphysical explanation. Its relief thus became a legitimate object for medical attention even if that relief was not accompanied by healing. 'A new sensibility had developed which was dissatisfied with the world not because it was dreary or sinful or lacking enlightenment or threatened by barbarians but because it was full of suffering and pain. Progress in civilization became synonymous with the reduction of the sum total of suffering. The result is a tendency to see pain as essentially a passive happening inflicted on helpless victims because the toolbox of the medical corporation is not used in their favour.' 'Medical civilization tends to turn pain into a technical problem and thereby to deprive suffering of its inherent personal meaning.' In Illich's assessment, current medical attitudes to pain have profound political overtones. Pain has become 'a social curse and to stop the masses from cursing society when they are pain stricken, the industrial system responds by delivering them medical pain killers. Pain thus turns into a demand for more drugs, hospitals, medical services and other outputs of corporate impersonal care and into political support

c

for further corporate growth no matter what its human, social or economic cost'.

Illich says despairingly that 'medical civilization focuses primarily on pain as a systemic reaction that can be verified, measured and regulated'. 'Pain calls for methods of control by the physician rather than an approach that might help the patient to take on responsibility for his experience... Compassion turns into an absolute virtue. The person in pain is left with less and less social context to give meaning to the experience overwhelming him.' Illich even claims that this 'objectivization and quantification of pain has progressed so far that medical treatises speak of painful diseases, operations or conditions even in cases where patients claim to be insensible to them'. Illich gives no references and this statement, trivial and silly in itself, seems to me to suggest the weakness of his argument.

Illich is viciously against the displacement by 'pain killing on prescription' of what he calls the sense of inevitable suffering moderated by free access to analgesics. In condemning medical drug treatment he quotes approvingly a passage from Medical Essays, written by Oliver Wendell Holmes and published in 1883. 'Throw out opium which the Creator himself seems to prescribe, for we often see the scarlet poppy growing in the cornfields as if it were foreseen that whenever there is hunger to be fed there must also be pain to be soothed: throw out a few specifics which our doctor's art did not discover: throw out wine which is a food and the vapours which produce the miracle of anaesthesia and I firmly believe that if the whole materia medica as now used could be sunk to the bottom of the sea, it would be all the better for mankind — and all the worse for the fishes.'

Illich condemns the idea that medicine should try to relieve pain at any cost. His particular example is the extreme situation in which intractable pain is relieved by lobotomy, the effective destruction of part of the patient's brain. Such individuals can still be aware that they are experiencing pain but its emotional content is lost and they are undistressed. This freedom from distress is obtained at a cost which Illich believes is never worth paying. Illich mentions neither the fact that simple lobotomy for pain relief is now rarely if ever performed and that many, probably a majority among the medical profession, would agree wholeheartedly with his view.

Illich claims that if a doctor regards pain as a technical problem this makes him 'unable to acknowledge the question pain raises in the one who suffers' and 'leaves him exempt from responding to the person in pain with compassion'. This is such nonsense that I must say so right here without waiting for the end of the chapter. There are undoubtedly some doctors who do not and perhaps cannot respond to the person in pain with compassion. But for the most part they are people who would not respond to anything with compassion. They should not be members of the medical profession but that is another story. To say that they lack compassion because they believe that pain is a technical problem which ought to be relieved is ridiculous. For the most part doctors are fully aware of the anguish that this technical problem causes.

Towards the end of the chapter Illich is anxious to distinguish his position from that of the masochist. He does not want to inflict pain in order that those who experience it may feel pleasure. His ideal is the 'culturally ordered self management of unavoidable pains and minimum recourse to sedatives, narcotics and anaesthetics *in extremis*'. This seems to me to be an expression with which few doctors would disagree. The crucial words are 'unavoidable' and *'in extremis'*. It is in the precise interpretation of these where Illich and most members of the medical profession would part company.

Illich concludes his account of pain by describing the survivors of Hiroshima. Apparently they were made emotionless and pain-free by the shattering impact of the destruction and death around them. This emotionless state then progressed to depression and a crippling profound guilt at their own survival. Illich believes that those in whom pain is suppressed will ultimately become like the survivors of Hiroshima though he fails to explain how they will become aware of the anguish of others which will make them so guilty. His final words are 'Pain loses its referential character if it is dulled and generates a meaningless questionless residual horror. The suffering for which traditional cultures have evolved endurance sometimes generated unbearable anguish, tortured imprecations and maddening blasphemies. These were also self-limiting. The new experience that has replaced dignified suffering is artifically prolonged, opaque, depersonalized maintenance. Increasingly pain killing turns people into unfeeling spectators of their own decaying selves.'

When confronted with a passage like that there is a temptation to write 'Rubbish' and pass on. Illich is so determined to curse medicine viciously and effectively that he ends by being merely silly and by writing a passage which most people would dismiss as ranting nonsense. But obviously he believes that he is making a major point. He is in a long tradition of thinkers who have tried to understand the cosmic significance of pain and to interpret its value for man. In this tradition pain is the slave who rides with the Roman general at his triumph whispering 'Remember that thou are mortal'. Pain is the hair shirt that constantly reminds the devout that comfort is illusory and that we are living in a world full of distress and disaster. Pain is the constant pointer to our mortality which prevents us from living a purely pleasure seeking life. Pain is the stress which brings out in man all the courage and compassion which make the agony bearable.

There can be no doubt that many who have been through intense pain regard the self knowledge they acquired and the unknown sources of strength which were revealed as valuable gains. But very few given the choice of acquiring the self knowledge and experiencing the anguish, or being free of the pain and failing to gain the self knowledge, would choose the former. Still fewer having gone through the experience once would elect to go through it again. Pain is a great evil and should not be welcomed simply because some of its side effects are good. The evil is greater than the good. Because the good offers some slight compensation for the evil we should not be blind to the idea that it would be better to be without both the evil and the good.

Few would deny that many of the most dramatic examples of human courage, endurance and compassion have been the direct result of war. In peace there is much less opportunity for the display of those virtues. But I cannot believe that any sane person would say that we need war in order to provide a stage on which human beings can display their virtues. Yet this is almost exactly what Illich is saying about pain. Like war it is mostly evil but it does have some good side effects. We must therefore be careful not to eliminate pain because although that would eliminate the evil it would also remove the good.

I find it difficult to believe that Illich has had much experience of seeing people in pain. My own experience too is limited but as far as I can see the only pain which produces the favourable effects which Illich describes is moderate pain of relatively limited duration. Even that sort of pain does not bring out the shining qualities in everyone. Like war what it seems to do is to write large the character of the person as it really is. The few who are both strong and basically good react as Illich would like to think everyone reacts. The weak are at least temporarily almost destroyed and may become little better than unthinking animals. The bad become worse and more vicious, even less aware than usual of the needs of others. Severe pain, or moderate pain indefinitely prolonged, destroys almost everybody. Very few can survive with any degree of dignity and most are reduced to the level of the brutes. If Illich had watched many in genuinely severe pain I do not think he would write as he does. It is possible, on the other hand, that he himself or someone close to him has heroically managed to endure such pain with dignity. If so, he is so impressed with the achievement that he cannot see that most people are incapable of surviving such horror.

Elsewhere in the book Illich emphasizes strongly that man should be treated as Everyman and not Hero. Yet in this chapter he seems to be urging that Everyman should be Hero. In the film Lawrence of Arabia, early in the war Lawrence (who would either have got on well with Illich or quarrelled furiously with him) is playing with matches and slowly extinguishing the flames with his fingers. A soldier watches him fascinated. Noticing that Lawrence's face does not flinch the soldier tries to do the same thing and shouts 'It hurts. What's the trick?' Lawrence replies 'The trick is not to mind that it hurts'. Illich wants us all to be Lawrences but unfortunately (or indeed perhaps fortunately) it is just not possible.

The fundamental point of Illich's thesis is that even if evil is avoidable we should tolerate it if a side effect of the evil is good. This seems to me to be a major error. Because pain is so valuable Illich believes it to be an essential part of human experience. If that is so then it is damnably unfair that it should be so unevenly distributed, that some people should live pain-free lives and drop dead suddenly at the age of eighty while others should be continuously anguished and die in great pain at fifty. It is one of the great myths that those who suffer are nicer and better than those who do not. If pain really is as important as Illich believes then surely we should be careful to inflict pain on everyone in order that all may experience its value. Illich claims that he is stopping short of this point but he is perilously close to it and is arguing in a tradition which has produced some who have not hesitated to go beyond it. If on the other hand, pain is basically an evil which very occasionally leads to some good, then we should do all we can to relieve the pain without the cant of saying that it is a valuable experience. If the balance between good and evil in pain is in favour of good, then we should attempt to ensure that everyone experiences severe pain in equal measure. If the balance is on the side of evil, then we should not hesitate to try our utmost to relieve it in those who experience pain in excess, with no nonsense expressed about the value of the agony.

For Illich the main answer to pain is to experience it in the context of a culture which explains its cosmic significance. This enables the sufferer to understand what is happening to him and supports him in his anguish. This is an extraordinarily sophisticated concept, far too extraordinary to be appreciated by most people in pain. Yet again Illich seems to require Everyman to have Promethean qualities. Traditional cultures differ radically in their interpretation of just what is pain's cosmic significance. Even within the Western Christian tradition pain presents enormous difficulties as witnessed by the many books on this topic full of extraordinarily contorted reasoning. There is certainly no consensus among Christian theologians as to what is the 'correct' interpretation of pain. Since they differ so radically from one another and are often mutually incompatible, most traditional interpretations must be at worst completely wrong and at the very best only partially correct. Most ordinary people confronted with the bitter experience of severe pain are not easily satisfied by traditional explanations even if they are backed by the whole culture.

Yet again the weakness of Illich's historical sense is revealed. He continually writes about traditional cultures as though they sprang fully armed on to the scene and will never change until they die. He displays little feeling for the idea that concepts of pain in any culture must have arisen slowly from primitive beginnings. There is no reason whatsoever for believing that in any culture this gradual evolution has ever stopped at a point of perfection. He does not seem able to consider the possibility that Western industrialized society may already be a traditional culture and that its account of pain is at least as valid and supportive as any other.

Because Illich is so narrowly concerned with man, he fails to go back to a point before man came on the scene and to consider the implications of the fact that pain is a universal phenomenon in the animal world. I am fully aware that Illich, like most people, believes that the conscious consideration of the meaning of pain is a strictly human activity. He may be right although the evidence is perhaps not nearly so strong as is often assumed. Nevertheless the phenomenon of pain must have existed for millions of years before man evolved. It must therefore have a universal biological function and it cannot have lost this function in man. This is not to exclude the possibility that contemplation of pain by man may help him to understand his place in the cosmos. But the validity of that contemplation can hardly be helped if the thinker deliberately ignores or worse rejects the fact that pain has a universal biological role as well.

I fail to see why Illich is so much against the ideas of Descartes and his successors that the purpose of pain is to warn the animal body that something is wrong. Once the warning has been given and taken note of, either by a reflex response or a conscious course of action, the value of the pain has disappeared. It should therefore be relieved if that is possible. This biological interpretation seems to me to be far more understandable and culturally supportive to the individual in pain than is any one of the traditional interpretations. I can see no evidence whatever that this active, sensible approach to pain in any sense interferes with the compassionate response of others to the sufferer. My own direct experience of some relatively primitive cultures and my historical knowledge of the great religions leads me to suspect that the reverse is true. It takes one a long time to become accustomed to the fact that in some parts of the world the usual response to disaster and physical anguish is laughter on the part of the observers. Because traditional cultures could do little about pain, because their conception of the consciousness of others was often very limited, in most societies until very recently, pain was ignored. Indeed it was often gratuitously inflicted without any thought of cosmic significance or compassionate response.

In the medical response to pain there is less to criticize than there is in most other areas of medicine. The idea that pain should be relieved whenever possible seems to me to be compassionate and to fit both with basic common sense and with a biological understanding of the fundamental importance of pain for living creatures. Of course doctors are human and some fail to be compassionate. Of course patients are human and a few respond to the idea that pain should be relieved with demands that all pains, even the trivial ones of a cut finger or a bruised leg, should be pharmacologically dealt with by qualified medical practitioners. But the majority of doctors and the majority of patients do not respond in this way.'I believe that our current cultural attitude to pain comes close to being as compassionate and meaningful as it is possible to me. Illich's stridency in this area worries me. He seems to have been so carried away by his theoretical arguments that he has become incapable of making a balanced assessment of the true state of affairs.

Having stressed the importance of our experience of and response to pain, Illich shows a curiously inconsistent response to its pharmacological relief. He damns in the strongest possible terms the modern medical use of pain relieving drugs. He uses to support his argument a quotation nearly one hundred years old in which a famous literary doctor condemns virtually all drugs except opium, alcohol and anaesthetics, all strangely enough used to abolish or relieve physical pain or to dampen the intensity of the emotional accompaniments of that pain. He seems to regard as important the obvious falsehood that opium and alcohol have always been used. Because they have always been used they should therefore be freely available for the layman to use for pain relief without medical intervention. Man had to learn to use alcohol and opium and many would say that his education has to date been inadequate. If opium were freely available it seems to me unlikely that it would not be widely abused for the relief of moderate pain for which other modern drugs are available. Illich seems unaware that the opium-based susbtances are still the most potent pain relievers in the doctor's armamentarium. Modern developments in pain relief have primarily led to the development of drugs of intermediate power which allow the potentially dangerous narcotics to be reserved for situations where they are truly necessary. As elsewhere Illich's major reform proposal seems likely to produce a considerable aggravation of the situation he wants to avoid, dependence of people on drugs and medicine in the widest senses of the use of these terms.

Illich does not seem to understand how most doctors react to pain. It seems to me that what might be called the orthodox position is something along the following lines:

1. Pain is primarily a signal that something is wrong with the body and is a stimulus to both patient and doctor to find out what is wrong.

2. Until the pain has been carefully studied and characterized it should not be relieved since premature relief may lead to mistaken diagnosis.

3. If possible the pain should be relieved not by analgesic or anaesthetic drugs but by removal of the cause.

4. If immediate removal of the cause is not possible and the pain therefore continues, because the pain has then ceased to have a biological function it should be relieved.

5. As far as possible pain should be relieved by relatively simple drugs such as aspirin which do not deaden consciousness and which leave emotional responses effectively intact. Illich nowhere mentions such drugs and writes as though he were unaware of their existence.

6. Only if the simple drugs fail, or if the situation is such that experience indicates that they will fail should the more powerful opium-like substances be used. They seem to be effective because not only do they reduce biologically detectable pain, they also deaden consciousness and reduce the emotional impact of pain.

On the whole doctors are criticized more for failing to provide adequate pain relief than for doing so in excess. There have been several recent accounts in the medical journals, written by doctors who have been patients, which describe the inadequate pain relief offered. Doctors are often unduly cautious in what they prescribe. To me Illich's attitude to pain seems to be much less compassionate and understanding even than this. By his advocacy of the traditional remedies of alcohol and opium his approach seems more likely to lead to overuse and abuse of analgesics. He bemoans the loss of the traditional cultural support for the patient endurance of pain in Western industrialized nations. He seems to want to reimpose it but that is not possible. We, perhaps unfortunately, have to start from where we are now and not from some hypothetical point in the past. Illich's attempt to reimpose a traditional culture is likely to leave society simply bewildered. In my opinion he hopelessly overestimates what that traditional culture did for and meant to ordinary people. No attempt in any culture to explain the cosmic significance of pain makes much sense other than to believers of high intelligence. In contrast the idea that pain is an essential warning signal is a simple concept which can be understood by anyone. It is part of a newly emerging culture which in its attitude to pain may well be more supportive than anything which has gone before.

Illich makes much of the compassion which is supposed to have permeated traditional culture. He provides remarkably little evidence for the common existence of such compassion and I suspect would be hard put to find much. There is at least as much compassion in our Western industrialized society as in any traditional culture. Our sins and our carelessness should not be minimized but to say that traditional cultures performed better than we did is a travesty of the truth. One has only to read accounts such as 'Akenfield' of what it was like to live in a traditional society even in benevolent England to realise that most people had little to lose but their chains. Our particular problem is size. We do not know how to deal with it and we are struggling somewhat unsuccessfully to prevent our health institutions from growing into bureaucratic monsters. There is no doubt that compassion is more difficult in such a setting and Illich is right to draw attention to this.

I cannot understand the paradox of Illich's antagonism to the use of analgesics by doctors coupled with his willingness to make a drug as potent as opium freely available to everyone. He relies on the good sense of the consumer to limit its use to situations where it is really necessary. I cannot believe − and here I may merely be expressing a prejudice − that if opium were freely available it would not be much more widely used than at present and that control by laymen would increase rather than reduce the use of mind-obliterating drugs.

Illich's approach to pain seems likely to achieve the exact opposite of what he desires. It would reduce cultural support because it would deny an easily understood rational approach. The withholding of drugs by doctors would reduce compassion: strangely it is much easier to be compassionate in a situation when one knows one can do something than when one cannot or when one must refuse something which is available. Lastly far from reducing analgesic abuse, free access to potent drugs by laymen would sharply increase it.

8 The Invention and Elimination of Disease

In this chapter and the next Illich gives lengthy accounts of the development within Western culture of attitudes to disease and death. He makes it very clear that he approves of many things in the past and does not approve of the point which history has now reached. What he does not make clear is the precise point at which he would like history to have stopped.

Illich points out that prior to the 16th century disease was usually regarded as dis-ease, a sickness of the whole man. Those who cared for sick people (and they were very few apart from immediate family and neighbours) responded to the sick man as a whole and not just to that portion of him which was ill. Sick people were usually cared for within their own community. Hospitals were the refuges of the destitute, pest holes where treatment of the inmates by the custodians was frequently appalling. There was remarkably little evidence of Illich's traditional compassion. Therapy had virtually no part to play. The hospitals were simply septic tanks where the destitute sick went to die; and where they often did so more quickly than had they remained outside.

Attitudes slowly changed and Rousseau and the French Revolution had a dramatic impact, presenting ideas which were the flowering of traditional concepts. These were then to be submerged and did not achieve dominance again until our own time. Rousseau, with his concept of the noble savage and his ideal of the primitive state, believed that the natural condition of man was healthy and that in his natural condition most diseases would prove self-limiting and easily controllable. Little care would be required that could not be provided by simple measures of love and attention by the patient's own family. Illness of the modern type was seen to be largely a consequence of a fall from a primal natural state.

The French Revolutionaries accepted these ideas with enthusiasm. Much as the state is supposed to wither under communism or as the total burden of ill health was to be reduced by the British National Health Service, in a genuinely free and equal society the need for doctors and hospitals would largely disappear. People would be much healthier, most sickness would be self-limiting and easily handled by the family or for those without relatives by local voluntary organizations. Only the incurable, the mad or the aged would have to be looked after in hospitals.

But in the first half of the 19th century these ideas were steadily lost. With increasing equality, instead of losing what small control it had over sickness and sick people, the influence of the medical profession gained ground rapidly. One of the most important developments was the recognition that there were far more diseases than had previously been imagined. The great burden of disease did not simply consist of the pest, the pox, the stone, fever and trauma but was of many different types each with its own cause and appropriate treatment. It was during this period that the idea of a disease which was quite separate from the patient and which could be treated without considering the needs of the patient as a whole developed. Illich condemns the change in diagnostic attitudes but cannot help but admire the magnitude of the intellectual achievement. Prior to this revolution 'sickness was still personal suffering in the mirror of the doctor's vision. The transformation of this medical portrait into a clinical entity represents an event in medicine that corresponds to the achievement of Copernicus in astronomy: man was catapulted and estranged from the centre of the universe'.

Illich is obviously uneasy here. He understands that the recognition that there were many diseases was a major achievement which opened the way to rational treatment and without which any fully rational approach to therapy was quite impossible. But on the other hand, this advance also opened up the possibility of considering a person's disease apart from the person as a whole. Although he does not explicitly say so, the tenor of his writing suggests that Illich finds this possibility so abhorrent that he would rather not have the achievement. He seems to ignore the fact that this recognition of the true nature of disease enabled the whole man to be treated more effectively and with more compassion than ever before. People tend to be embarrassed by and to turn away from those for whom they feel they can do nothing. If one can do something practical to help compassion tends to flow much more easily.

Illich seems to be ignorant of much of the more reflective writing in medicine. One of the strongest themes running through the writings of doctors from the early 19th century to our own time is the need to treat patients as whole people who happen to have a particular disease, and not just as cases of that disease. Medical journals have readily published accounts by outsiders of how doctors should treat patients. Thus, John MacMurray wrote in the Lancet in 1938 'The patient as a person requiring help is the focus of all problems in medicine. If medicine treats diseases, then a classification of diseases into bodily and mental will arise in which the unity of the person is lost sight of.' The fact that there is so much writing along these lines indicates that the profession itself saw the danger very early on and has constantly striven to counteract it though by no means always with success. Illich may be right in his impression that undesirable attitudes are now burgeoning as never before but he should recognize that many members of the profession feel much the same way.

Illich has opinions about the uses of measurement in medicine similar to the ones he has about the classification of disease. He does not like statistics and uses the results of statistical studies capriciously. He points out that one of the first successful uses of statistics was Cotton Mather's demonstration, in Massachusetts in 1721 that people who had been inoculated were indeed protected against smallpox. He does not condemn directly but by implication when he also says that Cotton Mather 'is better known for his inquisitional competence during the Salem witch trials than for the spirited defence of smallpox inoculation'. Illich is hinting that there cannot be much right about statistics in medicine when one of its founders was a witch hunter. He does not seem to accept that few men's lives are consistent and all of a piece and that especially when new ideas are growing, inconsistencies abound.

Paralleling changes in attitudes to disease were changes in attitudes to hospitals. From being pest houses they first turned into museums of disease where doctors and students could learn to recognize the various patterns. They then became experimental laboratories for treatment and finally, as some of the experiments began to bear fruit, places where healing actually begins to take place. Again Illich hesitates to condemn the change outright but the phraseology he uses shows that he thinks little of it. 'The pesthouse has been transformed into the compartment-alized repair shop.' The very success of the transformation in hospitals has opened the way for the removal of much disease from the responsibility of the family and the local society. Again because of the possible end products of this process Illich seems to condemn the success instead of taking the attitude that it must be applied with compassion and common sense. He is an expert simultaneous disposer of baby and bathwater.

Another broadside is delivered against the idea of the normal. The concept that there are many factors in a patient which can be measured, that some of these factors tend to show a characteristic pattern in those who subjectively feel well and that they show deviations from this pattern in those who subjectively feel ill, arouses Illich's ire. This is because it has many times been shown that some of those patterns observed in those who are subjectively ill can also be detected in those who are subjectively well. Doctors have therefore begun to tell people who are subjectively well that they are objectively ill. Illich feels they have been so successful that no one now knows whether they are well or ill without going to a clinic to find out. 'Society has become a clinic and all citizens have become patients whose blood pressure is constantly being watched and regulated to "within" normal limits.' Illich has a point but again he fails to emphasise how much the medical profession is itself concerned about whether a measurement which differs from normal should lead to a recommendation for treatment. In most cases the answer as yet must probably be a cautions 'No' since we do not know whether the deviations are caused by, are causes of or are merely associated with a disease. Only in the second case will treatment alleviate or cure the disease: in the first and third cases attempts at correction will do no good and may cause harm. Illich's choice of high blood pressure is singularly unfortunate. This is one of the few situations where a clear deviation from normal is an indicator of almost certain subjective disease to come. And moreover the disease that will come is not trivial: it is a stroke, a heart attack or a slow failure of the kidneys or heart. And drug correction of the deviation leads to a return to normal or near normal susceptibility to strokes and to chronic heart and kidney failure, though not as yet to heart attacks. This is one of the few unequivocal examples where treatment of a subjectively well person because of an abnormal measurement offers clear benefits.

Illich does not even have any kind words for the group of people — among whom Laing and Szasz are perhaps the best known — who have themselves constantly attacked the idea of normality with regard to mental function. They have asserted that mental disease is what physical disease last was in the 18th century, a disease of the whole person. Moreover in most cases this disease is an entity with no existence apart from that stemming from the preconceived attitudes to normality on the parts of the medical profession and the lay public. In Illich's eyes the sin which Laing and Szasz and the others have committed is to admit unequivocally that mental disease is different from physical disease and that the medical model of sickness is valid in the latter but not in the former. They have 'rendered it more and not less difficult to raise the same kind of question about disease in general'. Their protests legitimatize the non-political status of physical disease. For Illich who believes that even physical disease is politically dependent this is a betrayal of the worst sort, a true 'trahison des clercs'.

Having disposed of men whom the naive might have thought would be his natural allies, Illich moves to his final condemnation of modern medical attitudes to disease. 'Industrial society cannot function without providing its members with many opportunities to be diagnosed as suffering from real, substantive disease as a distinct entity. An over-industrialized society is sickening in the sense that people do not fit into it. Indeed people would rebel against it unless doctors provided them with a diagnosis which explains their inability to cope as a health defect. Diagnosis transfers the reason for the individual's breakdown from the engineered environment to the organism which does not fit... Until sickness came to be perceived as an organic or behavioural abnormality the patient could hope to find in the eyes of his doctor a reflection of his own anguish. What he now meets is the gaze of an accountant engaged in an input output calculation ... (The patient is taught) only just as much as the doctor considers necessary to gain the patient's cooperation in his engineering of interventions and circumstances. Language is taken over by the doctors: the sick person is deprived of meaningful words for his anguish ... Iatrogenesis due to the doctor's control over the language of suffering is one of the major bulwarks of professional privilege. As soon as medical effectiveness is assessed in ordinary language, it immediately appears that most effective diagnosis and treatment does not go beyond the understanding that any layman can develop.'

The doctor who fails to recognize that there is a good deal of truth in these words, no matter how much they may be exaggerated, has little insight into his own profession. But the basic description of medicine's response to illness is much more profound than Illich would admit. Change the emphases slightly and it is a splendid description of the ways in which all societies in all ages have responded to illness. Traditional cultures always put the blame for illness on the individual (sin, or deviations from the society's mores) or on some outside agency (avenging God or malevolent spirit). No traditional culture has ever admitted the organization of society to be at fault even when it is easy to demonstrate that, say, the method of sewage disposal is altogether wrong. Our own society has progressed a long way: in contrast to the traditional cultures its members continuously question the value of its methods of organization.

The idea that compassion is a characteristic of those in all traditional societies who regard themselves as healers is a nonsense which is sharply contradicted by any experience of most such societies. It is true that logic and 'cold' thought (would 'hot' thought be any better?) are applied by modern doctors more than by the healers in any other society or their predecessors in our own. It is true that some people rebel violently against this, none more effectively than D.H. Lawrence in his poem 'When I went to the scientific doctor' (page 45). It is also true that the cold thought produces more effective medical intervention than has ever before been possible and that such logical or cold thought in no way prevents the doctor from responding to the patient's anguish. It simply means that he does not have to cover the incompetence of his medicine by the excessive warmth of his emotion. Illich must have been singularly unfortunate in his contacts with doctors.

Illich's comments about language are, of course, completely correct. Doctors do use language to deceive and to mystify, not only patients but students and each other. However it is naive not to realise that here, for once, the modern doctor is following in the hallowed footsteps of the healers in traditional cultures. Obscurantism and mystification have always been the major − often the only − sources of power of the healer-priests. The difference between them and modern medicine is that the power is now real and therefore there is no need for the obscurantism. Illich is right on the mark in arguing that if medicine is to be made more responsive to the needs of society it must use ordinary language whenever possible.

Illich claims that most of the treatments which even he admits do more good than harm have two characteristics: they are cheap and they can be self-administered without medical intervention. When talking about common diseases he is largely correct but he fails to understand the reasons for this and again confuses causes and consequences. The methods he is talking about were initially neither cheap nor capable of self-administration. The cheapness and the possibility of self use did not cause the remedy to be effective. Instead the effectiveness of the remedy and its usefulness in a common disease led to its manufacture in bulk leading both to cheapness and to constant refinement and simplification so that it could be administered on a large scale without a great deal of training or experience. Illich's understanding of the sources of change, development and success in medicine is gravely defective. Most ineffective treatment is complex and inevitably becomes more and more so as unsuccessful attempts are made to refine it. When no method is successful almost every doctor has his own approach and the complexity and the dogmatism are bewildering. But effective treatment does arise out of this highly unsatisfactory situation. Eventually some experimental procedure does work unequivocally well and the process of simplification and cost reduction begins. Progressively all the ineffective traditional procedures are eliminated until one is left only with the simplicity. But the simplicity never just happens. It is the consequence of long-continued development in a medical context.

In most cases the same is true of the cheapness. Few remedies are inherently cheap and simple. The low cost comes from the continual refinement and from the possibility of mass production in the case of remedies for common diseases. Even so the question of cheapness and simplicity with effectiveness is by no means universal. Many diseases are not common. Although in sum the number of those suffering from all uncommon diseases is huge, the number suffering from any individual one may be very small. In this case even with highly effective remedies economies of scale cannot be applied and treatment may always be very expensive. But would it be truly compassionate to eliminate work on unusual diseases just because not many suffer from them and because any treatments likely to be discovered are almost inevitably going to be expensive? There are undoubtedly real problems in this area which have not been solved. Governments are reluctant to finance research on rare diseases because there are few votes in this area. Pharmaceutical companies are equally chary because, even if success in finding a remedy is total, profits will always be small. It seems to me an area where the finance must come from either Government or private philanthropy and where a little hubris must be used to push through schemes which could not be financially justified.

In other situations it has to be recognized that techniques can never be cheap and simple. To open a patient's chest, take over artificially the roles of the patient's heart and lungs for a while and to repair a defect in that heart is never going to be the sort of procedure which Bob at the corner shop could handle. Yet again are we so governed by cost-effectiveness that we cannot devote such extravagant resources to a few who will unequivocally benefit from them?

But in spite of Illich's defective understanding of the ways in which effective remedies develop, he is unequivocally correct when he argues that the profession is unduly restrictive about the administration of many of the treatments which are both cheap and easily administered by people of only moderate intelligence. In this situation doctors can retain exclusive professional use only by mystification and by the invocation of almost non-existent complexities and dangers. The performance of abortions in very early pregnancy and the administration of such drugs as oral contraceptives and antimalarials should undoubtedly be removed from exclusive regulation by the medical profession. Of course occasional disasters will happen but they do now when the procedures are under medical supervision. Most of the disasters come out of the blue and it is difficult to see what medical knowledge could prevent them. It should not be beyond the wit of a cooperative profession to devise a swift and effective back up service in these situations. The excess danger of having these remedies more readily available would then be negligible.

Illich does dismiss too easily some of the arguments against self-administration of treatment as opposed to administration by doctors or even by non-medical personnel. It is silly to deny that sick people are often inevitably very emotionally involved and find it difficult to make rational decisions. If one is making a technical decision about therapy one requires the greatest possible objectivity. This is simply not possible to achieve with self-administration in most cases. Sick people are often the easiest victims of the patent medicine manufacturers. Removal of professional control would inevitably increase this type of exploitation and I believe that some controls are necessary to protect sick people both from themselves and from commercial interests who would exploit them.

Illich's panacea for current medical problems is what he calls the deprofessionalization of medicine. It is often difficult to nail down precisely what he means by this but in the last paragraph of the chapter he gives a useful summary. He begins by saying what he does *not* mean:

1. That specialized healers should disappear.
2. That genuine competence should not be utilized.
3. That there should be no exposure of malpractice.
4. That public funds should not be used for medicine.
5. That modern medical techniques should not be used.
6. That specialized medical assistance should not be available to the newborn, to accident victims and the dying.
7. That medicine should not be evaluated by public scrutiny.
8. That the state should protect individuals against practitioners of medical cults even if these should embody all that is worst in modern medicine.

On the whole I am inclined to heave a sigh of relief. What Illich does not mean seems to me reasonable with the exception of the last point. My own view, and I suspect that of most doctors, is that some form of sanction should be available for use against those who mislead the public irrespective of whether they are professionally qualified or not or of whether they are using public or private funds.

My relief is much less apparent when it comes to the list of things which deprofessionalization does mean.

1. A bias against the mystification of the public. No reasonable person could disagree with this but it is important to recognize that modern medicine uses this technique less than any traditional culture.

2. A bias against the mutual accreditation of self-appointed healers by which is presumably meant that doctors themselves should not decide who is to be admitted to the ranks of the profession. This is a real problem area. I can understand clearly why Illich feels this way but so long as entry to the profession is regulated by competence in technical courses and examinations, it is difficult to see what other method may be used.

It is possible that much argument in this area is directed at the wrong point, the actual temporal moment at which some form of licence or degree is awarded to the new doctor. In Western industrialized societies the failure rate in medical schools is so low that for practical purposes the individual becomes an accredited members of the profession at the time of admission to medical school. It is much less difficult to envisage non-professional participation in the selection of medical students. As I shall discuss in the last chapter, I believe that current methods for medical student selection are seriously in error and that the profession does need to set its house in order or other systems of outside involvement will rightly be devised. However I have even less confidence in such potential external schemes than in the present methods and this is an area where genuinely constructive internal reform could have a dramatic influence in changing the whole character of the profession for the better.

3. A bias against public support of and legal discrimination on behalf of medical guilds. The meaning of this is not entirely clear and its inter-pretation must differ from country to country. But it is true that to date public bodies have often agreed with what doctors recommend, that sometimes these recommendations have been in the interests of the profession rather than the public (though usually well dressed up as the latter) and that this type of situation is beginning to be exposed. Again I would prefer the profession to reform itself. Like Illich I am doubtful as to whether it will but I have not completely lost hope.

4. That public funds used for curative purposes should be freely available to all and not administered under the prescription and control of doctors. But they must be under the control of someone and it is not obvious that Illich has any sensibly clear ideas on this. I certainly cannot envisage any new structure being put into operation by any Government which would not further increase bureaucratic if not medical control of the public.

5. That no professional shall have the power to lavish on any one of his patients a package of curative resources larger than that which any other could claim for his own. I am not sure what Illich is getting at but if he means what I think he does then no one should ever be treated for haemophilia or for severe trauma or for kidney failure or by cardiac surgery because it would be quite impossible to give everyone these facilities if they should require them. This seems foolish and certainly lacking in compassion for those whose misfortune it is to have an illness which cannot be treated cheaply. If taken to its logical conclusion in all areas of life — and Illich consistently makes it clear that he is using medi-cine to illustrate general principles — then this attitude inevitably leads to a denial of excellence and individuality. Illich continually protests his

belief in the value of these but I sometimes wonder about the depth of his commitment. I occasionally suspect that benevolent dictatorship rather than genuine democracy would be his preferred form of government — provided that he is the dictator. Apart from anything else, this preoccupation with expense would almost certainly prevent the development of any new cheap remedies. For example, Illich on several occasions writes of penicillin with approval. Yet the first patients treated with penicillin received it at a cost which was truly astronomical. The same is true of insulin and of almost any drug. It is only when efficacy has been demonstrated and mass production becomes appropriate that most remedies can become cheap. In the early stages of development it is usually impossible to say whether a drug or a technique will be genuinely effective or not. Illich's approach would cut off the good and the bad alike.

6. That tax funds should not be used to finance the more costly kinds of technical devices. Again a blanket refusal seems ridiculous. Should we really not finance a fully effective technique which at relatively high cost saves lives which would certainly be lost without it? How can we be sure that a device which seems very expensive initially will not become much more economical? Nevertheless medicine is undoubtedly vulnerable on this point. It has gone overboard for tehcnology and much of it is of little value. But, contrary to the usual interpretation, the problem is not an excess of scientific zeal but a lack of it. It is an odd fact that while drugs are exposed to rigorous controlled testing before they are released, surgical procedures and technical devices may not be. There is much room for improvement and this again will be dealt with in the last chapter. At this point I should just like to say that it is sometimes the lay-controlled sources of finance which have been most irresponsibly lavish and it is the lay members of ethical committees who are most reluctant to authorise controlled trials of any new technique or procedure. They are the ones who often believe that if it is new it *must* be better and that it is therefore unethical to compare in a scientific way the new with the old.

7. It means the unmasking of the myth according to which technical progress demands an increase in the specialization of labour, increasingly arcane manipulations and an increasing dependence of people on access to impersonal institutions rather than on trust in each other. I agree with much of this provided it is recognized that with complete validity techniques can go one of two ways from their inception. Some become more and more sophisticated and if they are to be used effectively do require more intelligence, education and skill. Others do become simplified and medicine has been seriously guilty in its failure to recognize this.

9 Death Against Death

In this long chapter Illich makes clear how fascinated he is with death. He starts with the boldly dogmatic statement that 'in every society the dominant image of death determines the prevalent concept of health'. He uses this dogma as the excuse for a detailed account of changes in the idea of death in the Western world, fascinating in its historical detail but of uncertain relevance to modern medicine. He describes the main stages through which man's image of death has passed and emphasizes that from a beginning as a concept free of medical associations death has become almost completely medicalized. As in the previous chapter Illich constantly implies that ideas of death were in the past distinctly healthier than those held today but nowhere does he state clearly what historical image is his ideal.

First death was seen as the result of evil action by some outside agency, sometimes human, often not. This was followed by the idea that death came as a consequence of God's action, not necessarily male-volent. Death then became accepted as an inevitable part of man's nature not caused by the active decision of an outside agent. In the 15th century instead of being simply a consequence of external action or of man's intrinsic nature, death became personified as an independent agent. 'From a life-long encounter death has turned into an event of the moment.' Instead of being, like God, immanent in history death has become a transient event, an interruption in the sequence but neverthe-less an event which books of the time indicate was of overwhelming significance. Illich says that it was at this time that it became important to die well and with dignity although this is surely a very much earlier concept. It was at this moment that medicine began seriously to enter the arena. 'Medical folk practices multiplied, all designed to help people, to meet their death with dignity as individuals.'

One of the doctor's functions was to work out when death was in-evitable and when it was not. The aim was to help nature, either to speed healing or to hasten an easy death. The doctor had no role to play in resisting death.

However also at about this time when death came to be widely accepted as a natural phenomenon, the way was being opened for consideration of the human body as simply an object. The corpse, which hitherto had been sacred and treated with little less respect than the living body, became simply material. Prohibitions against its use or disposal, for dissection for example, began to fall away.

Francis Bacon was the first to begin overtly to question the idea that man's death came at an inevitable time and place. He wrote that one of medicine's functions, instead of assisting Nature and easing death, might be to fight against Nature to prevent or delay death. This concept gained ground rapidly and before long it began to be believed that everyone had a right to a full and active life with a medically-regulated death at the end. Originally this idea was primarily held by the bourgeoisie but it was taken up by labour unions and related groups. Before long 'everyone', instead of including only the educated middle and upper classes, really did mean everyone.

Illich then makes some fascinating asides about the power of old men and their success in creating childhood in order to keep their young weak and under control. Although he does not draw the parallel this idea certainly has relevance in current medical education where, with little justification, in many countries postgraduate medical education is being made more and more prolonged.

The final change in the concept of death began in the 19th century when medicine began to lose the simple distinction between sick and well and started to label everyone as suffering from a specific disease. Death then completely lost any personified or unitary status. It simply became the consequence of a specific disease process which if it could be understood, could always in theory and sometimes in practice be prevented. For the modern doctor death always has a cause and therefore in theory can always be avoided. Illich emphasizes that this concept of medical control over death gives immense power to the doctor, and equally obvious that the power is largely illusory. In spite of intense medical effort the life expectancy of those who reach sixty-five has changed little over the last half century. Many more people reach sixty-five, but despite a few successes in limited areas medicine is still almost impotent in the face of death in the aged. But so potent is the myth as opposed to the reality that it is considered abnormal to die except under careful medical control.

Illich points out that the current situation is associated with many serious problems. It means that the doctor's presence or influence at the death bed has become more all pervading than that of the priest in a traditionally Catholic country. The regulation of life and death has been handed by society to the doctors even though their power in this area is largely illusory. Death without a medical benediction is an indignity which must be avoided at all costs. In order to illustrate medical attitudes to death Illich tells a story which I find difficult to interpret. A woman tried to shoot herself but succeeded only in lodging two bullets in her spine leaving her almost totally paralysed. A surgeon whom Illich claims to know kept her alive by heroic measures and 'considers her case a double success: she lives and she is totally paralysed so that he no longer has to worry about her ever attempting suicide again'. I do not believe that the surgeon meant anything of the sort when he spoke to Illich. He might have made some bitter comment about the value of his work but I am very doubtful as to whether the comment represents the considered judgement of the surgeon concerned. The irrational and maliciously vindictive side of Illich's attitude to medicine seems to show itself here.

Illich claims that the nearly universally believed but largely erroneous idea that medicine can save lives prevents people from getting worked up about 'murderous environments foisted upon man by the Industrial State. Medicine, not religion, is the new opium of the people'. This is exaggerated nonsense and again illustrates the way in which Illich feels free to be inconsistent in order to score a point. He fails to note that doctors have been at the forefront of the fight to clean up the environment and also that in an earlier chapter he has railed against those whose aim is to try to eliminate environmental health problems.

One consequence of the fact that death is now no longer seen as simply an inevitable consequence of being man but as always the result of some cause, is that there has grown up an attitude which seeks someone to blame for death. Death is no longer something which must be accepted in as dignified a way as possible as a part of man's humanity. Death is now always someone's fault, a technical failure on the part of medicine or its organisation. There is a good deal of truth in this and the approach is at least partly responsible for the rise in medico-legal problems in North America. However it should not be forgotten that the idea that death is *never* anyone's fault but is a consequence of being human has been the battle banner of the obscurantist incompetents who from the time of Semmelweiss to the present have used it to cover their inadequacies. As so often the truth lies at neither extreme but only in a common sense middle way.

In this chapter Illich repeatedly gets carried away and blames medicine for the most extraordinary things. He says that the claim that everyone has an equal right to a medical death has been used to expand dependence of everyone on a limitlessly expanding industrial system in general and on medicine in particular. 'Revolution, repression and even civil and international wars are justified in order to defeat the dictators or capitalists who can be blamed for the wanton creation and tolerance of sickness and death.' Illich really is splendid in his unparalleled ability to ride off madly in all directions at once. A few paragraphs previously medicine was the opium of the people, now it is the catalyst for revolution and war. Medicine is certainly used in the propaganda both of those who would repress and those who would revolutionize but Illich surely cannot be so naive as to believe that this is anything more than a cloak for quite other aims.

One of Illich's best points is his criticism that death has become more and more hospital orientated with death outside hospital frequently being considered a failure of the system. The idea has grown that hospitals are the places where seriously ill people can best be treated. Since those with life threatening disease are obviously the most seriously ill, equally obviously most people believe they must die in hospital. No one can seriously doubt that this is an area where medicine has gone wrong. There is a case for death in a hospital environment where facilities are available which are present in few homes, but for older people at least there is little to be said for the present system of death under the sort of intensive care which would be appropriate for someone who had just had a major operation. There are people in medicine, such as those involved in the hospice movement, who are struggling to make death within an institution a dignified and fully human affair and their influence is increasing. Nevertheless this is a problem which requires urgent attention. If possible death should take place at home and, if not, those working in institutions to which dying people are taken must substantially rethink many of their attitudes.

While the ideal of hospital death is debilitating and destructive enough in an industrial society whose whole philosophy is accustomed to it, it is doubly destructive when applied to traditional societies. Individuals from such societies transferred to a hospital may literally find their personalities disintegrating. 'People are deprived of their traditional vision of what constitutes health and death. The self image that gives cohesion to their culture is dissolved and atomized individuals can be incorporated into an international mass of highly "socialized" health consumers.' This is a major point and one where constructive thought has hardly begun. It is increasingly apparent that one of the most effective ways to destroy a traditional culture is to import medical aid, yet this form of aid is one which still meets with near universal approval among supposedly well-informed people in both donor and recipient countries. As so often Illich mishandles what could be a telling point by exaggeration and lack of rigour. He writes 'In many a village in Mexico I have seen what happens when social security arrives. For a generation people continue in their traditional beliefs; they know how to deal with death, dying and grief. The new nurse and doctor, thinking they know better, teach them about a Pantheon of evil clinical deaths, each one of which can be barred, at a price. Instead of modernizing people's skills for self-care, they preach the ideal of hospital death. By their ministration they urge the peasants to an unending search for the good death of international description, a search which will keep them consumers for ever.'

How many villages has Illich seen in this depth? How many generations has he lived in order to observe the process at work? How many doctors and nurses do actually preach the ideal of hospital death? Illich has the germ of a major point that Western medicine in traditional societies can do irreparable harm. The struggle against death which is a dominant factor in the life style of the rich is translated by development agencies into a set of rules by which the poor of the earth shall be forced to live. But Illich weakens his point by the obviously silly way in which he presents it. Nevertheless I believe it is one of the most important in the book.

This chapter is full of examples of silly or wrong comments made in pungent and effective language. Illich writes 'natural death is now the point at which the human organism refuses any further input of treatment. People die when the electroencephalogram indicates that their brainwaves have flattened out: they do not take a last breath ... Death has become the ultimate form of consumer resistance'. The facts about the electroencephalogram (EEG) are simply wrong. In the vast majority of patients, even for those within hospital intensive care units, the EEG is not used to diagnose death. Death does occur when a last breath is taken or when the heart stops. The EEG is simply a new and genuinely harmless device which is called upon rarely and only in a highly specific set of circumstances to assist the doctor in deciding whether or not death has occurred. This splendid polemical passage has therefore little basis in reality.

In this chapter Illich makes fundamentally valid points but he diminishes their impact by his preoccupation with past history and his extravagant language. Medicine is very destructive to traditional societies. Medicine has taken control over death and individuals have lost the right to decide with dignity how they shall die. Society forces man to abdicate decisions in this area to a medical establishment which has largely ceased to behave with any judgement or responsibility. Individuals are not regarded as human but as technical devices which must be kept going at all costs. What is needed is a return to the situation where doctors in consultation with the patient are prepared to take the responsibility for deciding enough is enough. But it is much easier for Doctor Everyman to abdicate thought and responsibility and to struggle blindly to the end. The hubris of Doctor Prometheus is required.

10 The Recovery of Health

This is a magnificent chapter. Many passages in it sound superb when read aloud. I have no doubt they have the capacity to arouse audiences to great enthusiasm. But like many a politician's marvellous speech the actual content is disappointing. The arguments set out in the earlier chapters are summarised. The fact that medicine is only one small part of the industrial enterprise whose hubris is leading to nemesis is made clear. One waits for the telling account of effective remedial action. But it simply is not there.

Illich begins by suggesting that man has had to cope with three frontiers, the attacks of nature, the attacks of his neighbours and the attacks of madness which come upon him when his dreams run free. Until recently myth has kept man from disaster on the third front but the myths have now been destroyed. Man has acquired the power to do things which previously were thought beyond his reach. And things beyond reach were the prerogative of the gods. Man has therefore committed the sin of hubris and nemesis is the inevitable consequence.

Industrialized and endemic nemesis

The basic problem is the dream of unbounded material progress, not just for a fortunate few, but for Everyman. The dream can be pursued vigorously and as in North America and Europe partly successfully but only at enormous and increasing cost. The price may not be worth paying if it involves total loss of individual autonomy and horrific destruction of the environment.

Many before Illich have recognized the problem. But almost all the answers proposed require increasing control, increasing bureaucracy and increasing industrialization. They can therefore never be successful in solving the basic ills which Illich identified. Only a deliberate winding down of industrial society with a progressive return to autonomous ways of existence offers any hope that man may be able to survive on earth indefinitely. If this does not happen Illich suggests that man will be able to survive only under a system of rigid superimposed controls which will make any current totalitarian state appear benign.

Medical nemesis

The world of medicine, Illich says, is only one example, though in some ways the most striking, of what is happening. The particular form of material welfare offered by industrialized medicine is the dream of Ambrosia, of unending, healthy life. The myth that this is achievable has been skilfully foisted upon society in order to ensure that more and more resources are devoted to medicine and more and more aspects of behaviour which hitherto were under individual control have been handed over to the doctors. The end result is a dramatic decrease in health in the widest meaning of that word as a result of clinical, social and structural iatrogenesis.

However, even if medical nemesis could itself be controlled, this would not prevent industrial nemesis since industry is now too powerful and some other aspect of industrial life would take over the power now wielded by medicine. Nevertheless medicine remains a worthy target for revolution. Medicine is a sacred cow and its slaughter might just be the event which triggered the end of the whole industrial approach. If individual control over health could be regained then individual control over many other things might also be recaptured.

From inherited myth to respectful procedure

In all traditional cultures the boundaries of possible human action were set by myths of various forms. Illich claims that these myths have now been destroyed and as a result man sees no limits to his arrogance. My interpretation of essentially the same facts is rather different. I very much doubt whether the myths really did hold man back from exploiting his environment. All they did was to justify the weakness and lack of power over the environment which man found all to obvious. As soon as it became apparent that man had the power to transcend what were previously thought to be absolute limits the myths collapsed. For perhaps two centuries man has behaved as though his power was absolute as though all problems were technically soluble, as though there were no limits. What seems to be happening now is that we are realizing that there are limits after all and that our power is not absolute. We are rapidly creating new myths, Illich's hubris and nemesis being an example, which are personifying what we already know to be the case.

Illich makes much of the newness of the problems which man must now face and of their unnaturalness. Again he implicitly hints that he is looking back to some ideal time in the past when society was perfect, and man was in a natural state. Of course this is a non-existent ideal. Man always has been and always will be an evolving animal both physically and culturally. He has coped successfully in the main with many potential and actual disasters. That does not necessarily mean that he will be able to cope with the one now confronting him. But the facts that the idea of indefinite material progress is now under vigorous attack, that new myths are being created to reinforce and popularise the limitations which are now obvious, give some hope that man will again prove flexible enough to cope. The coping may even be along the lines of which Illich would approve.

Illich is, however, very doubtful. He believes that sacred myths genuinely did limit man's actions in the past but he recognizes that it would be almost impossible to recreate such myths in a modern society which had the power to enforce limitation which man did not already instinctively feel. He therefore suggests that the only hope will be for humans to agree about basic values and procedural rules. Why he is more optimistic about the possibility of agreement on these points I am not sure. There seems to be precious little agreement on basic values in the world at present. And even in situations where basic values are agreed, procedural wrangling frequently seems to destroy the possibility of any effective action. To me it seems that the only hope is for unequivocal demonstrations with hard evidence that things are going wrong. This will then generate a will for change which will at first be expressed through existing institutions, then reinforced by myths. If these prove inadequate new myths will evolve. But the pace will inevitably be slow. We have to start from where we are and in the democracies at least we have to persuade many people that we are moving in the right direction. The situation may well get much worse before it begins to get better.

My own view is that the way to rapid reform in medicine is not through lay control of medical practice and medical administration. In my very limited experience it is laymen rather than doctors who have proved most vulnerable to the persuasions of the medical megalomaniacs and who have been instrumental in enabling a few influential doctors to inflict the excesses of industrial medicine on unsuspecting populations. An internal revolution within medicine seems to me to offer more practical hope of real change. There is no shortage of doctors who are beginning to think along these lines and in the last chapter I shall try to outline some possible strategies whereby change might be pursued. I regret that I do not have the faith that Illich has in the desire of most people to indulge in self care. Democratic lay control of the structure of medicine is likely to lead in the opposite direction. Ibsen may well be right and the only hope may lie with the hubris of a well informed minority within medicine who believe that Illich is basically correct in his assessment of what has happened to medicine and who are prepared to apply pressure to try to ensure that medical practices are restricted and changed. The clamour which in any democratic society follows any proposal for a reduction in expenditure on any social service suggests that this will be a task for heroes and not ordinary mortals!

The right to health

Illich begins this section with a brilliant summary of his thesis which deserves to be quoted in full.

'Increasing and irreparable damage accompanies present industrial expansion in all sectors. In medicine those damages appear as iatrogenesis. Iatrogenesis is clinical when pain, sickness and death result from medical care; it is social when health policies reinforce an industrial organization which generates ill health; it is structural when medically sponsored behaviour and delusions restrict the vital autonomy of people by undermining their competence in growing up, caring for each other and aging, or when medical intervention disables personal responses to pain, disability, impairment, anguish and death.

'Most of the remedies now proposed by the social engineers and economists to reduce iatrogenesis include a further increase of medical controls. These so-called remedies generate second-order iatrogenic ills on each of the three critical levels.

'The most profound iatrogenic effects of the medical technostructure are a result of its non-technical functions, by which it supports the increasing institutionalization of values. The technical and non-technical consequences of institutional medicine coalesce and generate a new kind of suffering: anàesthetized, impotent and solitary survival in a world turned into a hospital ward. Medical Nemesis is the experience of people who are largely deprived of any autonomous ability to cope with nature, neighbour and dreams, and who are technically maintained within environmental, social and symbolic systems. Medical Nemesis cannot be measured but its experience can be shared. The intensity with which it is experienced will depend on the independence, vitality and relatedness of each individual.'

This brilliant description, not I think of the present but of a possibly not too far distant future, should be impressed upon the mind of every doctor and everyone who has anything to do with any aspect of health services. It could happen. Unfortunately the last sentence is very important and I am not sure that a majority of individuals will hate what Illich sees as medical nemesis: they may actually welcome it.

Illich then goes on to say that at the moment there are only two possible courses of action: either society will become increasingly dominated and regulated and controlled by industrial requirements, with medicine leading the way, or society will accept quite different limits of behaviour, will destroy the influence of the professions and of industry and individuals will recover their ability to care for themselves, to amuse themselves and to learn for themselves.

In the last paragraph of this section Illich comes as close as he does anywhere to suggesting a possible programme for action. He recommends the introduction of legislation which will do the following.

1. Proscribe medical technology to professionals until those devices and means that can be handled by laymen are truly available to anyone wanting access to them.

2. Enable people to leave the industrial mode of existence and to live in a different way without being assigned a sick role by some specialist.

3. Abolish controls over addictive, dangerous and useless drugs and shift the full burden for their responsible use from the health professionals to the sick person and his family.

4. Prevent experts from defining what is healthy and recognize each man's right to define his own health.

5. Abandon standards of professional expertise in assessing health care personnel and allow popular choice to entitle elected healers to government-supported jobs.

6. Allow the communities served and not professional review organizations to assess the worth of health care.

When I first read this list I substantially lowered my estimate of the value of Illich's book. It seemed to me that he was interested only in destroying and not changing for the better and was proposing a list of things so unpractical as to render his judgement in all areas suspect. I am writing this after having read the book several times again and after listening for several hours to Illich speaking both in public and in private. The impression remains. He is interested only in total commitment to destruction and not in a controlled, critical but nevertheless basically sympathetic response from doctors.

The first proposal is silly. Illich is suggesting that no modern medical technology must be used by doctors until all the things that can be used by laymen are so being used. Apart from the problem of agreeing with government agencies — who may well be much tougher than the profession in this area — what techniques are suitable for lay use, this would impose an utterly illogical ban on all surgery, all intensive care after accidents, all diagnostic radiology and so on. If Illich believes that any society could agree to such a law he is dangerously out of touch with reality.

Points 2 and 4 are reasonably sensible although certainly in the democracies no legislation is needed here. The rights of individuals to drop out if they want to, and to define their own standards of what is healthy are nowhere in danger in the genuine democracies.

Point 6 is at least partly correct. Professionals should be involved in such assessment if it is deemed necessary because only they know how to ask the truly awkward questions and can detect misleading answers. But there is certainly a role for much greater involvement of lay personnel who may ask quite different yet very relevant questions which professional personnel might never think of.

Like point 1, points 3 and 5 are so silly and unrealistic that they brand Illich as being totally out of touch with reality. There are some publicity seeking charlatans within the profession and many out of it. The melancholy history of quacks down the centuries provides all too convincing evidence of the enthusiastic followings such people can generate. Legislation of this type would be a charlatan's charter and would lead to a gullible public being put in greater bondage than ever before.

Hygiene as a virtue

Although there are occasional lapses into meaningless rhetoric this last section of Illich's book is on the whole a sane and balanced view of what a truly healthy society should be and what should be the role of medicine in such a society. What is lacking is any realistic concept as to how we might get there from here. His main point is that the maintenance of health in the widest sense of that word depends on the conscious formation of enlightened habits. Again he seems to believe that at some undefined point in the past we were naturally healthy within the framework of a traditional culture. It would be foolish to deny how much we have lost of the best of some traditional cultures or to claim that our own society is in any sense healthy. But I personally know of no traditional culture in which any but a tiny minority could have been considered healthy in Illich's sense. Despite all their faults, if one assesses the ability of the modern democracies to ensure that most of their peoples live most of their lives in a reasonable state of well-being I doubt whether the performance can be bettered by any traditional society. It seems to me to be untrue to say as Illich does in his very last paragraph 'The true miracle of modern medicine is diabolical. It consists not only of making individuals but whole populations survive on inhumanly low levels of personal health.'

For me a much truer note is struck earlier on. '(The ability to cope with illness) can be enhanced but never replaced by medical intervention in the lives of people or by the hygienic characteristics of the environment. That society which can reduce professional intervention to the minimum will provide the best conditions for health.' In the last chapter I shall try to provide some practical suggestions as to how this goal may be achieved.

11 Proposals for Change

'The medical establishment has become a major threat to health.' In spite of all my criticisms of his work, in spite of all his exaggerations and inaccuracies, I still feel that Illich's first sentence is right. He is wrong about the current seriousness of the threat; he is wrong in extrapolating so glibly to the whole world from the countries of his own experience, he is wrong in his estimate of the contributions medicine has made. But he is right in his assessment that things are beginning to go badly awry and that action is required if they are not to get very much worse in the near future.

So I agree that the main thrust of description of the state of medicine and its relationship with society is not too far wrong. His description of the syndrome is reasonably accurate but his refusal to recognize that most of the critical material he has assembled comes from medical sources and that much of the work has already been done by doctors themselves is totally misleading. Illich is not such a lonely prophet as he imagines himself to be. He does not have a monopoly of insight. Joseph Conrad wrote a book 'The Secret Agent' which was first published in 1907. In it the Professor says to Comrade Ossipon with regard to the views of a third revolutionary 'And so Michaelis dreams of a world like a beautiful and cheery hospital.' Ossipon replies, 'Michaelis may not be so far wrong. In two hundred years doctors will rule the world. Science reigns already. It reigns in the shade maybe – but it reigns. And all science must culminate at last in the science of healing – not the weak, but the strong. Mankind wants to live – to live.' Many doctors here share Illich's concerns but there is little doubt that they are ignored by many of their colleagues or that their plaints fall on many deaf ears.

But while Illich is not too far out in his descriptions of what is now and what things might become, he is hopelessly wrong in his understanding of the pathogenesis of the situation. Despite his claims to be an historian, he seems to have little feel for history. Despite his concern for the individual, he seems to have little understanding of how ordinary people operate. Despite his repeated desire that the earch should be a place in which Everyman should live, he consistently wants his Everyman to be a Hero.

Illich has a view of the operations of the medical profession which is very close to the vision that John Kenneth Galbraith has of the functioning of the modern large corporation. Galbraith sees the corporation as deciding not what the public needs but what the corporation wants to supply. It has enough influence then cynically to manipulate public desires so that people feel a great hunger for this object which the corporation supplies. In a way almost exactly predicted by the corporation, the supplies are made available. The corporation makes a profit, it reinforces its power and influence and poor individuals in society are trapped ever more deeply in the machinations of the new industrial state.

According to Illich modern medicine operates like the modern corporation. It has decided that it wants to supply perfect health for everyone. It has cynically set about persuading people that that is what they want, and having created the desire, it has made arrangements to supply it.

To me this seems to be a completely false interpretation. As far as I can see health has always been a major concern of traditional societies. At no time in the past has the great majority of individuals felt able to cope with pain, disease and death in a sturdily independent way. Most people have always felt bewildered in the face of these trials and have always been willing to put themselves in the hands of healers and priests who have offered remedies and religions to enable man to cope. In many traditional societies the role of the healer priest is all pervading and crippling. So many rules must be adhered to, so many rituals followed if an individual is to remain healthy that sturdy independence is often non-existent. For thousands of years the healer priests have been as powerful as, or sometimes more powerful than, rulers in the communities they 'served'.

One thing limited their influence. That was their near total lack of success in treating disease and preventing death. Certainly some primitive remedies worked. Certainly healer priests, like many modern doctors, were willing to exploit for propaganda a spontaneous return to health which had nothing to do with their machinations. Certainly by means of mystifying language and impressive ritual many were persuaded that the healing was more successful than it really was. But never and nowhere were traditional healer priests consistently able to point to regular major successes in man's battle with disease.

Medicine had inherited the role of the healer priests. It is obviously heir to the healers of traditional societies but the 20th century collapse of much organized religion has led in addition to many people looking to doctors for advice and comfort which they previously received from their priests. It has therefore obtained a double influence. But much more than that, although it is less successful than it and the public think it is, it can point to a long series of spectacular and consistent miracles.

The conquests of polio and smallpox, the removal of parental fear that their children will die of pneumonia or diphtheria or tuberculosis before they reach adulthood and many other successes are unequivocal and readily demonstrable. Because of the traditional desire of the sick to put themselves in the hands of others, because of the obvious power of modern medicine, society has willingly accorded to doctors an influence and a power which they have never had before. But the profession has acquired this power in a fit of absentmindedness. On the whole it has not deliberately sought it, and it does not know what to do with it. Far from using it in a heroic and Promethean manner, it has bumbled along making decisions of enormous significance without realising what it is doing. In some ways this is far more dangerous than a cold and deliberate bid for power would have been.

Finally, Illich is tragically wrong about solutions and perhaps even uninterested in them. In some ways it seems that the last thing he wants is for medicine to be reformed effectively either as a result of internal or external influence. Instead he wants doctors to behave in a ridiculous and arrogant fashion in order to horrify people so much that the whole structure of industrial society, including medicine, is brought crashing down. Hence his solutions are unrealistic or trivial, quite impossible to achieve in any democratically organized society, yet incompatible with all but the most benevolent (and therefore non-existent) totalitarian regimes. Some of his remedies, as in the case with his ideas on pain and his desire to abolish all control of both doctors and quacks, seem likely to intensify rather than to ameliorate the very problems he discerns. While complaining all the while about the use of mystifying language by doctors, he and his disciples consistently write and talk in ways which are often nearly incomprehensible. Sir Karl Popper's remarks about the philosophers of the Frankfurt school seem to fit Illich and his friends. They are in 'a tradition which accepts that something is profound when it cannot readily be understood and that the sign of a man who has had a university education is that he can write and speak in a manner which is both impressive and incomprehensible'.

Some tentative suggestions

My basic philosophy of the way to bring about political change at any level in any society consists of two propositions. The first is that we must start from where we are and we cannot do that unless we can see our present position with a reasonable degree of realism. The second is that, without any exceptions at all, the consequences of any proposed change are always different from those that the proposers predict. The gap between expected and actual consequences becomes greater the greater the degree of change proposed. Since almost invariably the consequences are less favourable than expected, the greater the degree of sudden change, the greater is the shortfall between hope and reality.

At the moment I think that both Illich and the medical profession have an imperfect grasp of reality. Many doctors do not realize how serious the situation is and only partly understand the origins of those defects in the system which they do perceive. Illich has a better but exaggerated perception of the current situation but has almost no insight into its origins. He has performed a service by taking the writings of some concerned doctors and setting them out in such explosive and inflammatory language that the ideas must command some attention. It is up to the doctors, infuriated by Illich's rhetoric, not to condemn him unthinkingly but to consider seriously his thesis, to admit where he is right and then to set about doing something about it.

If a large enough number of doctors does become sufficiently roused to make a realistic assessment of the state of medicine, what is the best way of generating change? Illich's answer is essentially to remove most controls and to allow the public to decide what it wants. He does not believe that the profession will ever be able to make the decisions to move medicine towards what he sees as a more favourable state. I think he is totally wrong. The thirst for miraculous health is such that lay opinion is likely to be captured by effective publicists anxious to acquire more and more power. The last state will be worse than the first with a public dominated more than ever by health concerns and unable to make any rational assessments of the irrational complaints of competing healers.

My own belief is that most doctors are neither particularly humane nor particularly perceptive of the needs of society in general or of patients in particular. But one of the strengths of medicine is that it has repeatedly produced great healers who have seen the necessity for reform and who have dragged along their colleagues, grumbling and complaining furiously, but nevertheless ultimately being willing to change. Often the great men have been successful simply because they have pointed to the ideals of the Hippocratic Oath and have shamed their colleagues into agreement. The agreement has not come from the heart but the hypocritical head. However as C.D. Darlington has noted when speaking of the early Christians, 'Within the community, they established a stern uniformity of conduct, a deference to their own rules. Now although such public deference must always engender private hypocrisy, it is in practice the only weapon invented by man for raising the conduct of a heterogeneous society above the average genetic and instinctive level'. Because of their claims to be possessors of high ideals no matter how hypocritical such claims may be, if doctors are to retain public respect they will always be vulnerable to those who demonstrate that the medical profession is not acting in the interests of society. Ultimately, if the idealists are persistent enough, they will always be able to force doctors to act hypocritically and grumbling and groaning, to surrender personal privilege and wealth in the interests of humane medical practice.

I therefore think that because of its supposed ethical basis the medical profession is vulnerable to enlightened pressure. But if it is to be fully successful such pressure should come from within and should be well informed. Ignorant outside pressure will always be angrily resisted.

Medicine is in a serious state and is in need of reform. But reform is likely to be effective only if the proposals are based on realistic information about the current situation and about its origins. I therefore think that such reform can be effected only by doctors themselves, by doctors sensitive to the criticism of laymen such as Illich. But doctors should not be under any illusions. There is a serious breakdown in the relationship between medicine and the public and unless doctors move to do something realistic about changing their behaviour themselves, heavy-handed attempts at reform will come from outside. Because of the vulnerability of lay opinion to all that is worst in medicine, the end result is likely to be much worse than before. Precisely contrary to what Illich hopes, there will be more bureaucracy, more waste, more meaningless control and the public will be even more firmly in the grip of those who want to remove its independence and control its destiny.

Simply in order to demonstrate that my approach to medicine is basically positive I shall conclude by presenting very briefly some possible solutions. These can be given in outline only here and I would not wish them to be regarded as more than tentative suggestions. There are four main issues which must be faced.

1. Is there too much or too little science in medicine?
2. Is there to much or too little technology in medicine?
3. Is there too much or too little administration?
4. Is it appropriate that a profession which claims to be a vocation and to offer a most important service to the community should also be the best rewarded financially?

Science in medicine

With 'love' being the only possible exception, 'science' is the word currently most misused in the English language. It ought to be a criminal offence punishable by at least seven years course-work in political science or social science, to use it without some definition. In the current context I mean by science the attempt, using reasonably reliable methodology, to ascertain the truth about situations in medicine. I am fully aware that any pedantic philosopher — which I sometimes am when wearing another hat — can shoot that definition full of holes. I am also aware that anyone wearing an average man full of common sense hat will understand very well what I mean. The role of science in medicine is to attempt to get at the truth. When defined in this way it is difficult to see how anyone could object to scientific medicine.

But the fact is that many do object to scientific medicine. In the minds of many average men full of common sense there is a strangely illogical antithesis between a warm and humane approach and a cold, scientific one. I personally find it somewhat difficult to understand why falsehood and ignorance should be warm, while truth and knowledge should be cold. They seem to me to be very nearly independently variable qualities. However I happen to believe that what we want in medicine is not less science but more and so I had better explain a little further what I mean.

We do not know whether most of the things which we do to patients are better for the welfare of that patient than if we had done nothing at all. And on the whole we most of us prefer to remain warmly ignorant rather than coldly knowledgeable about the situation. It is I think obvious to anyone who looks at medical practice with anything like a critical eye that many of the things which are done to patients either have no influence on the outcome of the illness or may increase discomfort and hasten death. Much money would be saved and many patients would be better off if less medicine were practised. But which bits of medicine should be discarded? The only way to find out is by an effectively designed controlled trial in which the consequences of no treatment are compared to those of treatment. If more such well designed studies were performed, I have little doubt that many currently used treatments would be dropped and many proposed treatments, after careful trial in a limited number of centres, would never be widely introduced.

Unfortunately it is often difficult to persuade doctors — and in my experience much more difficult still to persuade most laymen — that to have a patient untreated may lead to an outcome more favourable than that resulting from any current treatment. The problem arises because of the illusion that in an untreated patient nothing is being done. Man's body is the product of hundreds of millions of years of refining evolution. Its survival depends on the ability of bodily control mechanisms to maintain the constancy of the physico-chemical features of the body fluids within which the cells are bathed. The potency of these mechanisms is extraordinary. It is only their superb effectiveness which prevents us from being continually surprised not that we get ill but that we ever remain well. In illness these internal control systems fight heroically against the agents which would upset their equilibrium. With any disease a massive effort is therefore continuously being made to counter the disturbing forces. Any human intervention will alter the balance of power in this struggle between disturbance and equilibrium. It is just as likely to hinder the equilibrating forces as the disturbing ones and it is therefore by no means self evident that any treatment is better than none. Yet while most people, both medical and lay, can see the validity of this argument, most also have great difficulty in overcoming their emotional conviction that to do something must always be better than to do nothing. It is this warm emotional conviction which has done more than anything else to encourage the introduction into medicine of damaging and ineffective methods of diagnosis and treatment. Only more and better science will perform the humane function of eliminating the errors encouraged by warm emotion.

Technology in medicine

Technology is a word misused almost as much as science and so again I must begin by attempting to define what I mean. In this context what I mean by technology is simply the application of a technique to a situation, without any critical consideration of whether the outcome is likely to be favourable or not. And while there is too little science in medicine in the sense in which I have used the word there is unequivocally too much technology. There is a certain type of doctor who is very impressed by techniques particularly when they involve electronics, computers and oscilloscopes: such doctors love flashing lights, rolls of chart paper and pale green lines on screens. So mesmerised are they by the complexity and cost of the equipment that for the most part they do not even begin to entertain the possibility that the expenditure of large sums of money on such wonders might fail to benefit patients.And so expensive and complicated techniques are introduced without any properly controlled trials. Since the desire to have such techniques available in one's own hospital or unit seems highly infectious, once one has been acquired they tend to proliferate hugely at enormous cost and with no real benefit — or at the very least before anyone can be reasonably sure that any real benefits will accrue to the patients. Techniques should be subjected to controlled trials at least as rigorous as those which new drugs must undergo. Only if the outcomes of such trials are favourable should the techniques come into common use. This very simple device of the application of more rigorous scientific standards would stop at the outset the introduction of much useless new technology. But if such a reform comes about it will have to be pushed by doctors since laymen seem appallingly vulnerable to the megalomaniac intentions of those members of the medical profession who are obsessed by the ideas that any innovation is good and that there is a strong positive correlation between the effectiveness of a technique and its cost.

Administration of medicine

One of the greatest paradoxes of the organisation of any modern profession or government department is that while most people instinctively understand what is required of an effective administrative machine, the administration machines actually constructed seem specifically designed to be both very costly and highly ineffective. An administrative structure whose function is to serve the public should be so constructed that the maximum number of decisions affecting individuals are made in the shortest possible time by other individuals in whom the public has confidence. Yet most administrative reforms seem to succeed in ensuring that members of the public almost never meet fact to face in the first instance with a courteous and competent person who has authority to make real decisions. Furthermore, the decision making process is so dominated by complex committee structures and tiers of organisation that even trivial questions may take months or years to sort out. The aim seems to be to set out a procedure which takes care of every possible circumstance and as far as possible eliminates individual error by eliminating individual responsibility. The result to the individual member of the public is a faceless and inhuman monster with which it is impossible to argue or fight. This leads to an apathy and a despair about the place of any individual in a modern bureaucratic state.

Medicine is no exception to this general picture. In all countries, irrespective of whether medicine is state or privately financed, the numbers of people with no technical role as health professionals but with purely administrative duties have increased. It is unfortunately true that the increases have been most dramatic in countries with state controlled systems and that the resulting administrative patterns have become labyrinthine and self defeating. It would be foolish to deny that changes in the pattern of administration have made some things better. But most of these things have been better for the professionals than for the public. There is an alarming tendency for improvements to be made purely for the benefits of administrators and to be in the interests of neither doctors nor patients. If our altruism has not been stirred by administrative monstrosities which obviously make things more difficult for the patients it is just possible that self interest may rouse the profession when the monstrosities make things more difficult for the doctors as well.

It is very easy to be uselessly generalised in one's comments on this situation so I shall try to be more specific.

1. It has several times been noted that the best administrators are those busy and competent people who hate administration. They are the ones who will make efficient decisions with the minimum of waffle and bumbling because they cannot afford to waste their time in unproductive ways. This means that as far as possible power should be in the hands of those people, whether lay or professional, who have no time to waste because their main function in life is not administrative. It also means that we should cease the ridiculous practice of defining promotion in a professional group as an opportunity to become an administrator. Once anyone becomes a full time administrator, no matter what their training, they cease to feel the same pressures to get things done quickly and effectively and they become infected by the administrative disease. As few decisions as possible should be in the hands of those whose function is purely administrative.

2. Attempts must be made to keep every medical institution as small as it is possible to be. The supposed increases in efficiency which come with centralisation and size have almost all proved either to be illusions or to have been gained by paying a price which ought to have been recognized as unacceptable. A good example is the closure of small hospitals in communities and the increasing centralisation of facilities in monster institutions. This has arisen because of a failure to recognize the extraordinarily simple fact that patients are in hospital for very different reasons. A surprising number are in hospital not because of any technical services which the hospital can provide but because, for reasons which have nothing to do with medicine, it is not possible for them to receive the minimal nursing care which in a well run 19th century middle class household they would normally have received at home. This sort of patient can readily be housed in an institution which essentially provides hotel facilities with no resident medical staff, no complex laboratory or radiological facilities, few professionals of any kind, but many people, often with no training at all, who are interested in looking after people. This sort of 'cottage hospital' is excellent for what it aims to do. It is cheap to run, it is usually close to the community it serves and it is often capable of generating a huge amount of community loyalty which is a major asset in helping to make it a humane place in which either to work or to be a patient. Above the cottage hospital should be another type of hospital whose function is to provide relatively simple technical services for those who are acutely ill. This requires simple operating theatres, radiological and laboratory facilities, resident medical staff and good trained nurses. Again because there are no facilities which most of the patients in hospital will never use, the institution can be kept small and can retain a good deal of

community loyalty. Finally there should be specialist hospitals in big cities which will take only that tiny fraction of patients who can be cared for neither at home nor in the other types of hospital. Only in these units would the full range of complex techniques be available. Only these hospitals would cost to run per bed what many of our big general hospitals, most of whose patients could be in simpler institutions, cost today. The effect of this type of structure would be to return most hospital facilities and hospital patients to their own communities and to reduce costs sharply since the complex facilities instead of being provided for everyone in hospital would be used only for those who strictly needed them.

3. We must assess much more carefully the levels of training actually required to enable people to do jobs effectively. The greater parts of most courses for most health professionals cannot be justified either on grounds of technical or general education. All that most courses do is to delay the emergence from childhood to adulthood on the part of the students, to reduce the number of years a person can spend in productive work and to increase the distance between the haughty qualified professional and the poor bewildered patient.

In essence all I am doing is stressing that Schumacher's slogan 'Small is Beautiful' applies to things other than economics. Doctors, with their long traditions as independent individuals, able to take their own decisions, must resist vigorously attempts to make them cogs in a supposedly smooth running administrative machine.

Medicine and money

One of the most interesting features of *Medical Nemesis* is Illich's consistent refusal to make the most of the attitudes of doctors towards money. This is partly because he feels that the personal accumulation of wealth by doctors has an impact on the factors with which he is concerned which is relatively trivial. But it is also partly Machiavellian. Illich quite specifically and quite deliberately says that he does not want to control medical racketeering. Such obviously anti-social behaviour constantly reminds the public that their gods have feet of clay and seriously limits the power of the profession. If all doctors were humane and not particularly rich their power as a profession would be enormously increased.

I am antiquated and hypocritical enough to believe that a profession which is as satisfying as medicine, a profession which continually makes public pronouncements about caring, should not be, as it is in most countries, a certain road to wealth and security. There is something offensive in the fact that doctors are on the whole extremely rich by any standards other than those of their immediate peer group. If Illich really wants to rouse the public against medicine, I personally believe he is being far too Machiavellian and that his strategy will fail. It is going to be very difficult to persuade laymen that doctors are as lacking in miraculous powers and even in competence as they in fact are. It will be much easier to arouse anger by pointing out the discrepancy between the high ideals which doctors often profess and their personal life styles.

But if Illich does not attack the groin in this way, others certainly will. Doctors must be made to realise the extent of their insensitivity on this issue and must stop being so greedy before it is too late. I am not optimistic of their ability to see that this really is an issue which could bring the whole pack of cards tumbling, and that if doctors do not reform themselves, someone from outside will most definitely do so. It should not prove impossible for professional bodies to set reasonable standards of fees and payments and to police these relatively simply. Unless something like this is done, the bureaucratic government machinery to carry it out will certainly be imposed in almost every country.

ACTIONS AT VARIOUS LEVELS

In all countries, while doctors are progressively losing to laymen their rights to make decisions they still have a good deal of power to regulate their own affairs. Possible reforms are legion and each country will have to devise its own. But I do not want to duck the issue of attempting to make specific recommendations concerning desirable changes. As I have stressed I believe that real improvements in the way we run a democratic society come from making small piecemeal changes in things which are obviously wrong and not from devising grand theoretical strategies for total revolutions whether bloodless or not. If the attitude of doctors is such that they are fully prepared to recognise problems and are eager to make effective changes, no matter how small those changes may be, the whole attitude of the profession towards the public and the public towards the profession will undergo a transformation.

I envisage changes being made at four main levels, of the individual doctor, of the organisation of the profession, of the relationship between government and medicine and medicine-related industries and of the medical school which is at least partly responsible for the face which medicine will bear in the future.

Individual doctors

The arrogance of some doctors faced with their patients is almost unbelievable. Yet alarming numbers of doctors are either unaware of how arrogant they are or being aware are unconcerned. I am not sure how their attitudes can be changed, perhaps by a confrontation with an articulately angry patient, perhaps by an effective novel and perhaps not at all. It may be that fundamental change in the area will require a change in the sorts of people who are admitted to medical school. But one can always hope that with maturity will come an ability to treat as equals patients who do not happen to have specialised knowledge but who, because the illness is happening to them, deserve a full and unpatronising explanation of what is happening and what the alternatives are.

One very practical thing which in most countries would change the attitudes of people to doctors overnight would be a change of heart on home visits. I have recently moved from a country where home visits are a major, though declining, part of medical practice, to a continent where home visits are almost unknown. In Britain much of the residual affection which is attached to doctors depends on an experience with a competent and humane individual who came to see a sick person in his own home. In North America much of the growing resentment against doctors is related to their near total refusal to leave their offices to see any sick person. When two people have to meet, who travels to see whom is a statement about a number of things, but in part about who at that moment is the more important. In North America the view in the profession is near universal that the doctor is always the more important, that the doctor should waste as little time as possible in traffic jams, that there are no circumstances in which the patient is more important than the doctor and that therefore it should always be the patient who makes the journey, no matter how sick he may be. This surely is hubris of the worst possible sort and together with doctors' wealth may well be the issue which could bring nemesis. If they are not to be destroyed, if they are to retain their proud traditions of humanity and concern, doctors must change their attitudes to home visiting. Sometimes doctors may be more important and sometimes the patients must travel. But sometimes, and especially with the old and the very young, it is the doctor who should make the journey. Even if the direct clinical results may sometimes be scanty, even if the patient is not so ill as was imagined, home visits are very frequently gains for both doctor and patient. In my opinion one of the touchstones of the real motives of any doctor should be the attitude to home visiting. I feel uncomfortably sure that in North America at least most doctors would be found to be something less than pure gold.

The profession

The professional bodies in each country are in a position to make decisions and recommendations which can be enormously influential in changing professional attitudes for better or for worse. Unfortunately such influential decisions are rarely made by men and women who know what they are doing and who are fully aware of the enormous consequences. Decisions which later turn out to be of seminal significance are frequently made by incompetent small men with small concerns, only interested in balancing the personal power games in the organisation concerned. As a result medicine has drifted disastrously with few attempts at leadership and far sighted thought. It is certainly not hubris, but a total lack of it which has been the problem in many cases.

One major positive contribution which professional bodies could make is to stop assuming that anything which improves the personal financial position of their individual members is necessarily in the interests of the profession as a whole. What is good for General Motors is not always good for America and what is good for individual doctors is not always good for medicine in relation to society. If doctors as a group set out scales of fees and remuneration which were not legally binding but made publicly available and therefore carried a good degree of moral weight, and if those fees were such that doctors were adequately remunerated but not at a level which consistently made them the richest group in a nation, then, as Illich fears, the profession would gain enormously in respect and in its ability to influence the future direction of medical care systems. But if medicine consistently behaves as a purely self-seeking, money grabbing profession then sooner or later it will be recognized as such and treated accordingly.

Professional bodies should also be much more prepared to get involved in making hard hitting recommendations, as fully as possible based on hard science, as to the real values of treatments and diagnostic procedures. These should concentrate on demonstrating which techniques are useful, which are not and which are ones where more evidence is required. Some effort should be made to channel some research funds into effective testing of this type and some pressures should be devised to ensure that individual doctors at least take note of the research findings. The pressures should always be moral and never absolute since expert recommendations may sometimes and perhaps often be wrong but as far as possible doctors should be discouraged from using techniques or drugs whose value is uncertain or harmful. The profession must become less obsessed with technology and with innovation for innovation's sake and must try much harder to prevent fashionable and irresponsible misuse.

Governments and medicine

Since even in countries where medicine is basically privately financed, much of the cash flowing into medicine ultimately comes from government or is dependent upon government decisions, and decisions made by government can be enormously influential in determining which way medicine will go.

On the whole and this is perhaps a hopelessly optimistic concept, government should operate on the ideas that small is beautiful, that centralisation is very frequently inefficient, that administrative 'reforms' should never lead to an increase in the number of administrators relative to those of technical and professional staff and that costly high technology innovations should be fully evaluated scientifically. Clearly it would be silly in a book of this type to make specific suggestions for specific national situations. All I want to suggest are principles which should guide those who are trying to influence the relationships between medicine and government.

One interesting way in which governments could influence things would be to change patent laws in an imaginative manner. At the moment drug safety regulations and patent laws are such that it is impossible for a drug in most countries to enjoy more than a few years of patent protection while it is on sale to the public. Patent protection is given equally to drugs which are genuinely much better than existing ones and to those which are no better or even worse. Since the period for which patent protection operates is so short, it is frequently the marketing skill of the company rather than the real effectiveness of the drug which determines whether or not a product is a commercial success. I suggest that while the basic patent laws should operate as at present, patent protection should be withdrawn from any compound which is not unequivocally better in some clearly defined way than existing compounds, before the new compound is marketed. This would sharply reduce the number of competing products and the incentives to market effectively drugs which have little therapeutic advantage. Simultaneously, drugs which genuinely do provide an advance should be given perhaps 30 years full patent protection, not from the date of the original patent but from the date at which the relevant regulating body (such as the Food and Drug Administration in the United States) gave permission for the drug to be marketed. This would reduce the often unseemly haste to market a drug before it has been fully tested, haste which often stems from the knowledge that patent protected time is running out because it is dated from the time of filing of the original patent. It would also enormously increase the rewards offered to genuine innovation and would reduce the current drug company emphasis on the need to market relatively ineffective products.

Medical schools

It is one of the illusions of both laymen and doctors that individuals
are admitted to the medical profession at the time they receive their
MD degree or its equivalent. The nature of the course followed and
the examinations set are supposed to determine whether people will
become doctors or not. This is an illusion because in most countries
the failure rates of students going through medical school are now
extremely low. For the most part people are selected to become doctors
at the time they enter medical school.

Another illusion is that the quality of a doctor five years after graduation is related to the content of the courses that the doctor took during
medical school and to the skill with which these courses were taught. It
is my prejudice that this too is a fantasy. These factors may perhaps
be important in the first year or two after graduation but by five years
their influence has almost disappeared and thereafter it is non-existent.

What then is it which determines what sort of doctor a person becomes? Only two factors are of any real significance. The first is what
sort of person *enters* the medical school. I do not believe that intelligence
and personality traits can be much altered by education after the age of
20. The second is whether the philosophy of the medical school emphasizes teaching or learning as the key educational process. This is becoming almost an anachronistic consideration since those which used to
emphasise learning have almost all been transformed into teaching orientated schools.

It is obvious to anyone who can see beyond the end of his nose that
no matter how complete and valid are the facts taught in a medical
school, those facts will be partly unknown to and partly forgotten by
even the best students within a week of graduation, will themselves partly
cease to be facts within a very short time and within 20 years of graduation will be of little value. After graduation, although occasional
'refresher' courses may be helpful, especially to morale, the only way in
which a doctor is effectively able to keep up to date is if he personally
seeks out selectively the information of value to him from a vast morass
which is available. One might have thought therefore that a major aim
of a medical school would be to help a student to prepare for a life time
of this sort of study, of learning for oneself. In the great majority of
the medical schools of the world nothing remotely like this happens. All
day, every day, students are fed ephemeral facts by techniques, ranging
from the traditional lecture to the modern computer, which will usually
not be available to them in their lifetime of practice. Virtually no sustained

effort is made to offer a different approach in which the student is set objectives and then largely left to find and to learn the relevant material by himself. Lip service to the concept may be paid during a brief elective or project course but compared to the sustained weight of teaching the impact is trivial. The end result is a doctor whose education has most effectively atrophied the only characteristics which would enable him to remain competent throughout a lifetime.

Can anything be done to improve the education system? I have serious doubts because the schools are now so permeated by experts whose raison d'etre is the provision of teaching rather than the creation of opportunities for learning that the problems of generating change are likely to prove unsuperable. The sort of change I would like to see would be for a medical school to set out for its students the objectives of the course and then to leave its students to tackle these objectives themselves. Formal courses would be provided for those who wanted them but they would be drastically reduced and positive efforts would be made to ensure that no student imagined those courses to be compulsory. Students learn in many different ways and they should be given the opportunity to use the ways most appropriate for them. For some lectures are ideal, for others (myself included) there is nothing like a good book, for others learning is impossible without a practical experience. Few if any medical schools allow this diversity to be expressed. Everyone is forced into the common mode of following time consuming courses and time available for learning is almost non-existent.

As to assessment I regret to say — or rather am pleased to say — that I regard examinations as essential goads and guides for most students. Examinations have innumerable faults: in this they are like democracy. Both examinations and democracy can appear to be extremely unattractive ways of doing things until one looks at the alternatives. *All* alternative methods of assessment are less fair to someone, whether teachers, students or patients, than humanely conducted examinations. It does no one any harm to be forced to make a reasonably realistic assessment of his own abilities using a technique which incorporates the minimum of purely personal bias.

In short the only curricular reforms I would like to see are the introduction of clearly stated objectives which are not dependent upon the personal whims of a single teacher, a drastic reduction in formal tuition with an emphasis on forcing the student to find things for himself, and a reasonable emphasis on examinations as a method of assessment. I think that students emerging from such a system would be rather less like shell-shocked morons than some of those who now emerge from our medical schools with the grandiose title of 'Doctor'.

But I have no illusions that any revision of medical education of this sort would have any substantial reforming effect on the profession. The Medical Schools would still continue to choose the students with the very best grades for entry. And all over the world these grades are now very good indeed and most would agree that medical students, when assessed by conventional standards are the cleverest of all students in most universities. There has been a dramatic change in the last twenty years. Before that medical students were certainly not the brightest of students: their stereotype was that of the cheerful games playing oaf rather than the studious intellectual with straight As.

Most medical educators pride themselves on the quality of their students. In my opinion this pride is largely misplaced. The students have succeeded in distorting the pattern of medical education. Instead of trying to decide just what knowledge and skills most doctors need — and coming to the blinding realisation of the obvious, that on the whole the practice of medicine requires a very modest intelligence — educators have allowed the intellectual abilities of their students to determine the nature of the education offered. As a result all concerned, students particularly, and to a lesser extent teachers and laymen have been dazzled by the idea that competent medical practice requires great intelligence. It has become impossible for someone of moderate intelligence to become a doctor. Yet the great majority of jobs in medicine do require only moderate intelligence and this disparity between the intelligence available and the intelligence required becomes a major source of distress and unrest. It leads to pressure for the creation of more and more unnecessary high powered posts and to the demeaning of those necessary types of work which should make up the greater part of medical practice. It also leads to very clever doctors believing that their rewards are not commensurate with their intelligence and hence to an increasing lust for material reward.

The idea that medicine is a vocation seems to be disappearing from our medical schools. Students want to get into medical school because that is the ultimate accolade for smart city-bred kids and their parents: they want to get into medical school because that is a certain route to wealth: and only very rarely do they want to get into medical school for those old fashioned vocational reasons. It is therefore not surprising that we are increasingly breeding a profession whose major concerns are academic empire building on the one hand, and the rapid accumulation of wealth on the other.

The bright students who go to medical school are not even particularly interesting. Their concerns tend to be narrow, their lust to get into medical school at all costs all consuming. Since coming to North America I have learned that a high proportion of students who want to get into medical school will stop at nothing at all in order to achieve their ends. Whatever the ability may be, it is inconceivable that those who will behave like this in order to get into medical school will ever make doctors who in any sensible meaning of the word could be described as 'good'.

I am therefore very gloomy about the current state of medical education. I see a cadre of narrowly intellectual, not very pleasant people, entering medical school and being herded through it in a way which is calculated to suppress any wider concerns they may have and to create a corps of brilliant morons, incapable of relating to their patients in any sensible way in spite of receiving more formal courses in sociology and psychology than ever before. Professor Stuart Sutherland of Sussex University in England recently wrote a book called 'Breakdown' in which he recounts in some detail his own breakdown and his encounters with those who profess to understand the working cf the mind. In the end Sutherland concludes that most students would learn more about psychology and sociology by reading great novels than by going through any of the courses now available. This conclusion would perhaps be unremarkable if Sutherland were not himself one of the world's leading psychologists. Unfortunately I do not see many medical students reading great novels and their ability to relate to people in a sane and helpful way seems to be almost inversely proportional to their theoretical knowledge of psychology and sociology.

Is there any hope at all for medical education and therefore for medicine? The people now going through medical school seem to me to be more likely than ever to create Illich's nightmare world in which insanely applied medical power dominates individuals to a greater and greater extent. I have little optimism that any reform of the educational process itself will lead to much improvement given the present types of student entering medical school. As I see it the only hope is to change sharply the characteristics of the people entering medical school. In Machiavellian terms this seems to me to be a possibility because the number of people governing the choice of medical students in each medical school is very small. If only one or two of these people begin to adopt radically different ideas about who should be admitted to medical school they may well be able to exert an influence out of all proportion to their numbers on the future development of medicine. If change is to be a possibility it seems more feasible to change the sort of people entering medical school than to change those who are already in it. The change will take place slowly but it will be much more profound than any other sort of reform.

I suggest that the first point to be recognized is that while medicine requires a moderate degree of intelligence it does not require superb intelligence. Most posts in medical practice can be more than adequately carried out by ordinarily able people. The available pool of adequate competence is enormously greater than the one which is now being tapped. For most of these posts an ability to get on with people in a reasonably sensible way, a determination to resist the wilder forms of academic idiocy, are much more important than very high intelligence. It therefore follows that what we should be looking for in medicine are moderately intelligent well-balanced people who want to be doctors not to prove their high academic ability, not to become rich but to fulfil what they feel as a vocation.

How are these people to be found? There is little doubt that at the age of 18 or 22 it is much easier to make a reliable assessment of academic ability than of personal qualities. The difficulties of making reliable assessments of people on the basis of a 30 minute interview have been emphasised again and again. Faced with these difficulties and obsessed with a desire to be fair to the candidates, medical schools have opted for the only route which offers any hope of any objectivity: they have selected those with the best academic records without for one moment asking whether in doing this they may be cheating not the candidates but the patients who will be treated by these super-intelligent doctors. It is at least arguable that medicine might in the long run be better served by deliberately and objectively selecting those with moderate academic records rather than those with the best. I am certainly not saying that no highly intelligent people are needed in medicine. Some certainly are required but this need could be met by taking far fewer into medical school than at present.

One way of being much more certain about personal qualities is to defer the selection process until much later, perhaps until the age of thirty after several years have been spent in jobs unrelated to medicine. What I would like to see is a sharp change in emphasis whereby at least half those selected for medical school are aged thirty or more and have had considerable experience of life outside the narrow confines of the medical profession. At this stage it is much easier to make a reasonably reliable assessment of personality and to select people who, while having more than adequate intelligence, have a genuine vocation and want to do medicine for reasons other than lust for academic power or a rich life.

What would be the advantages of recruiting a substantial number of medical students at this much later stage? The first, and by far the most important, would be to bring into medicine a group of people with a broad range of experience of life outside the medical profession. These people would bring to medicine perspectives quite different from those of the present doctors who on the whole have appallingly little experience of or interest in life outside medicine. They would have opinions of their own and would be far more resistant to attempts by their teachers to mould their opinions.

The second advantage would be that it would be possible for those governing medical school admissions, without losing any objective assessment of academic ability, to use other criteria as well. By 30 most people have given some indication of their true worth in non-academic terms and it would be realistically possible to choose people whose common sense, moderate and equable approach to life would enable them to handle effectively the great majority of jobs in medicine.

Thirdly admission at around age 30 would ensure that most of those admitted were neither academic empire builders nor interested in riches. With rare exceptions the megalomaniac academics have to start much earlier than that — and are fully aware that they have to do so — if they are to realise their ambitions. Those who at 30 are prepared to commit themselves to being students for four or five years are almost equally unlikely to be motivated purely by lust for gold. Such entrants would come into medicine with a healthily diverse group of motives and would bring to it aims which are rarely seen with the present method of recruiting.

There are two obvious apparent disadvantages, that these entrants would on the whole have a decade less of life to give to medicine and that they would require substantial rethinking of the courses in most medical schools. Both disadvantages are largely illusory. In most Western countries there is by any sensible standard no overall shortage of doctors. There are serious problems of distribution both in terms of geography and speciality with some regions and some specialities having a substantial excess and some a substantial deficiency of doctors. I submit that these problems of distribution are at least in part a consequence of our recruitment of the city-bred super-intelligent into the profession. As we choose such people more and more exclusively I predict that no matter what the overall numbers going into medicine, the problems of distribution will become progressively worse. I suggest that people of moderate intelligence, entering medicine a decade later after a much wider experience of life, are in contrast much more likely to solve the problems of distribution. It may well be worth accepting the missing decade in order to correct the distribution problem which with our present type of medical student is likely to prove insuperable.

The second disadvantage, that the medical school curriculum would have to be substantially rethought in order to meet the needs and demands of those more mature students is one which I personally do not see as a disadvantage at all. If it produced deep thought about the fundamental philosophy of medical education as opposed to the trivia of curriculum development it could do nothing but good.

MEDICAL HUBRIS OR MEDICAL NEMESIS

Illich believes that the present state of medicine is disastrous because of its iatrogenic impact on individuals and society. He sees that state as having arisen from an overweening pride and lust for power, a longing to make decisions and perform miracles which should be the prerogative of the gods. This hubris is the cause of the present impending nemesis.

I also believe that the present condition of medicine in its relation to society is seriously defective. I do not think that the situation is as bad as Illich would have us believe, but it is certainly bad enough. All trends suggest that things will degenerate progressively and that Illich's faulty description of the present may not be far wrong as a true account of the future.

But I disagree strongly with Illich's understanding of the causes of our present disarray. Doctors have acquired an empire in a fit of absent mindedness. They have inherited the positions of both traditional healers and traditional priests. But the potential power is much greater because in spite of the weaknesses doctors can offer miracles which are consistent rather than capricious. When coupled with the desire of most people for health and long life, it is obvious that the influence of the profession is potentially far too great. That influence has been acquired because it has been and is being thrust upon doctors. With rare exceptions doctors have not actively sought it. Because of the real power of doctors they have repeatedly made decisions whose impace on society is incalculable. They have unleashed forces which it may not be possible to control. But on the whole these decisions have been made by small men with small concerns, shuffling papers while sitting bored around a table in some dingy committee room. Doctors have not realised that they have been making decisions which should be made by the gods. Because of the medical profession's ignorance and narrow concerns it has not been guilty of hubris.

I personally would have been happier had hubris been one of doctors' sins. The gods are not going to intervene in the organisation of medicine and so whether we like it or not doctors have to make the decisions. It is time the medical profession became aware of what it is doing. Conscious hubris, a knowing involvement in decisions which will affect the structure of society in the deepest possible way is what is required. If doctors abdicate their responsibilities in a headlong rush to become Everyman, Illich's prophesies will come true. It may well be too late but some at this hour must still try to snatch the fire from heaven.

Index